Contents

Foreword

It is unusual to encounter a book on teaching and learning in primary care that takes the reader from the detail of how to arrange the furniture for effective learning in the consultation through to an elegant account of the theories that support the practical suggestions. But this approach mirrors the experience of general practice where mundane and dramatic events follow each other throughout the clinical day, observed and experienced through the lens of generalism and made sense of as a practitioner reflects on their meaning.

Changes in the healthcare system and differences between countries are important, but do not alter the fundamental truths of learning in the primary care setting. Learning to deal with common problems, to deal with uncertainty, to work with a team of other clinicians, to undertake illness prevention and health promotion, and to understand and value the differences between generalism and specialism are essential for competent and satisfying practise. This book provides a companion to learning about all of these tasks, but importantly it also provides a guide to the rigour and complexity that primary care teachers must themselves learn to embrace if they are to be effective.

Dame Lesley Southgate
Professor of Medical Education
St George's University of London
September 2005

Teaching and Learning in Primary Care

Richard Hays
Professor of Medical Education
Keele University, UK
James Cook University, Australia

Foreword by

Dame Lesley Southgate
Professor of Medical Education
St George's University of London

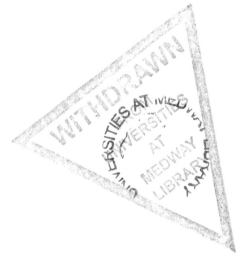

Radcliffe Publishing
Oxford • Seattle

Radcliffe Publishing Ltd
18 Marcham Road
Abingdon
Oxon OX14 1AA
United Kingdom

www.radcliffe-oxford.com
Electronic catalogue and worldwide online ordering facility.

First published by Eruditions Publishing, Melbourne, Australia. This edition is not authorised for sale in Australia or New Zealand.

British Library Cataloguing in Publication Data

A catalogue record for this book is available from the British Library.

ISBN 1 85775 756 4

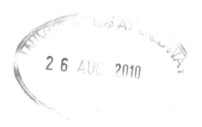
Typeset by Anne Joshua & Associates, Oxford
Printed and bound by TJ International Ltd, Padstow, Cornwall

Preface

This is the first edition of this book to appear under this name and be published in the United Kingdom (UK). It is an updated version of the original version which, while still highly relevant to general practice medical education anywhere, was set within an identifiably Australian context. Context poses challenges for authors of books about primary care, because healthcare systems even in the developed world differ most at primary care level. Differences include the level of training of the health professionals, the extent to which different health professionals must collaborate towards common goals, career pathways, remuneration, and management and governance structures.

While not attempting to describe in detail the various contexts in which general practice education is delivered, this edition attempts to recontextualise the content into a broader, primary healthcare team approach, more like that found in many healthcare systems. The focus is still on educational principles and maximising learning within primary care, and these principles should be very similar in many healthcare systems. Although published primarily in the UK, the educational material is not embedded in the UK system – other books do that better. On the other hand, this book arguably focuses on teaching and learning better than those that focus on the structure of particular healthcare systems. Some readers may prefer to read both kinds of book.

In preparing this edition I was surprised to find how little has really dated. This may reflect the developments in medical education over the last three decades. The 1960s saw general practice and primary care become recognised as a clinical and then academic discipline. The 1970s and 1980s represent a period of substantial development in both curriculum and identifying the micro-skills required for apprenticeship and small group teaching and learning. The 1990s was a period of consolidation and development of more valid and reliable assessment methods, such that formal assessment during and at the end of training is now routine in most nations. The more recent focus has been on evaluation, accountability, safety and quality, mainly at the postgraduate level. While clinical governance and safety monitoring mechanisms are now more widespread, the pace of development in teaching and learning practices at the practice level has slowed. Hence the contents of this book are just as relevant now as they were when it was first released around six years ago, although materials have been updated as required.

Another cautionary note: this book was written not just for novice teachers, but also for more experienced teachers who want to delve a little into the education theory that underpins practice. The depth varies, but is sufficient for entry-level academics in primary care. Readers who are considering an academic career should benefit from the deeper discussions on curriculum, assessment and evaluation, while those who are not might choose to skip those sections. The main aim of the book is to be a practical guide for those involved in general practice supervision at the vocational training level, although the principles are similar for undergraduate teaching. Those more involved with medical students might gain something from reading the book *Teaching and Learning in Clinical Settings* (Radcliffe Publishing, 2006), which focuses more on undergraduate teaching and learning.

Richard Hays
September 2005

About the author

Richard Hays went into full-time rural procedural and then general practice for a few years before being asked to help teach GP registrars and medical students. He soon realised how little he knew about medical education, and then embarked on a career in academic medicine. He has both a PhD in educational psychology and an MD in medical education, and he has worked for 20 years in both postgraduate and undergraduate medical education, including establishing a new medical school at James Cook University in Australia. He maintains part-time clinical practice as well as teaching in both community and hospital settings. He has written several book chapters and books on rural health and medical education, and has published about 100 research papers. From early 2006 he is the Head of the new medical school at Keele University in the United Kingdom.

Chapter 1

From clinician to teacher

We live and learn, and big mountains are stern teachers.

Bill Tilman

Different role, different skills

Those invited to be supervisors are usually regarded by their peers as sound clinicians. They will be well-trained, experienced professionals used to providing healthcare to their patients in a comfortable environment which they control. Hosting learners in such a setting is a special, yet disruptive, experience for two main reasons. First, it inserts learners into the personal world of the supervising professional. Supervisors are now challenged, in almost every patient encounter, to reflect on what they are thinking and doing in front of both a junior colleague and their patients – a form of 'mental undressing' in public. This can be discomforting, but can also assist supervisors to keep up to date as questioning by learners often provokes supervisors to look up information related to patient care. Indeed, some experienced supervisors describe supervision as 'built-in continuing professional education'.

Secondly, hosting a learner in a practice inserts an 'outsider' into the many special relationships that exist between patients and their healthcare advisers. Here it is the patients who are mentally undressing before a wider audience, but with the expectation that their health problems will be dealt with competently and confidentially. Consequently there are ethical considerations to ensure that potential harm to patients is minimised. Patients must be willing participants, but even so judgements must be made about what it is reasonable for learners to do with patients.

Clinical supervision is a form of apprenticeship training, as learners gain from observing and doing things in the real world. The traditional apprenticeship systems have been based on time, or rather the duration of working together, in the expectation that knowledge and skills will, in time, pass from supervisor to learner. However, this reliance solely on time is now challenged by the combination of knowledge transfer, skills workshops and guided experience, which produces competent professionals faster than time-based experience alone. It is this more sophisticated approach that is now employed in apprenticeship training. The current trend is to focus on measuring the attainment of competencies when learners are ready, potentially accelerating progress in a more flexible way.

Nevertheless time spent with clinical supervisors is of critical importance, for two reasons. The first is that the key learning resources are patient interactions, and supervisors are the source of the patients. The second reason is that novice learners can learn a lot from observing and imitating (or not) what their supervisors do. This contact provides essential experience in the application of knowledge and skills gained elsewhere through reading, lectures and skills workshops. If we assume that it is better to learn without making mistakes that

1

might affect patient care outcomes, then guided learning is better than independent learning. Further, we now know that different learners have different learning styles and come to learning with different prior experiences and levels of knowledge. Learners vary in their capacity to absorb knowledge and master skills. Particularly where teaching is one-to-one or in small groups, good teachers must have the skills to recognise and work with learners who are on individual pathways to a common end-point.

This is a much more active process than simply allowing learners to observe what we do, yet few clinicians receive any training in the more active model of clinical supervision during clinical training. Instead, many fall back on strategies endured as students. Some of these were effective, others less so. Most of us can remember instances where we either observed or suffered humiliation at the hands of an imperious teacher, and we would try to avoid making those obvious mistakes. Similarly, many will remember inspiring teachers on whom we may attempt to model our behaviour. However, despite our perceptions of what might or might not work, even our personal experiences are not necessarily a good guide. Most of our teachers received no teacher training either, so modelling our teaching on them could see a repetition of the mistakes made by generations of clinical teachers.

Just as clinicians learn from clinical training, those who want to teach benefit from some teacher training. A critical question for teachers to ask of their work is: 'How have I helped this learner learn something faster or better than if left alone?' This book is written for those who want to answer this question.

The nature of general practice

A prerequisite to becoming an effective general practice clinical teacher is an understanding of the nature of general practice. This probably takes a few years of post-certification (Membership of the Royal College of General Practitioners, Canadian College of Family Physicians or equivalent) experience to acquire, but this is variable. The conceptual basis of the discipline could be summarised as being a social science that applies scientific knowledge in the real world. The principles of primary care medicine include:

- Provision of continuing, comprehensive care to a defined practice population. General practitioners (GPs) must be able to deal, at least initially, with any clinical presentation. Over a period of time, we collate in our memory and medical records substantial personal databases about patients and their contexts. Each time we see a regular patient, we have access to prior material and lay down more. It is analogous to having a full-colour DVD writer and reader in our heads; we can add another track for each consultation and can replay earlier tracks, particularly with access to well-constructed (and used!) patient records.
- Dealing with common problems. Other medical disciplines rarely have to deal with common complaints that are often regarded as trivial, but comprise a substantial proportion of our workload and cause substantial morbidity; for example, urinary tract infections (URTIs) and tennis elbow.
- Dealing with uncertainty. GPs work with a low prior probability of serious illness and disease. That is, most patients have self-limiting or slowly evolving

conditions, for which a delay in diagnosis makes little difference. Therefore, GPs tend not to investigate problems as thoroughly as hospital-based doctors do, and often 'use time' to allow disease to evolve and become clearer or improve. This approach has an inevitable error rate, and one of the skills of general practice is to minimise diagnostic and management errors through recognition of early departures from normal pathways.

- Illness prevention and health promotion. Increasingly, GPs are seen as powerful agents for educating patients about living healthier lifestyles and for ensuring vaccination and screening programmes are implemented appropriately. This role has been assisted by computerised recording and recall systems, often with targeted funding that rewards achievement of targets or penalises failure to achieve those targets.
- Management skills. Increasingly, GPs are expected to be managers, not only of their own practices, which are really small businesses, but also of healthcare for their patients. Models of local GP organisation now exist in several nations to improve coordination of GPs with each other, other health professionals in primary care, and with secondary and tertiary care. In the United Kingdom (UK) this role is arguably provided by primary care trusts (PCTs), although the relationship is more complex because PCTs are also commissioning agents for healthcare services. However, few GPs have received any formal training in either business management or healthcare management. The most relevant time to learn about management is during postgraduate training.
- Education skills. Throughout the world, medical schools are turning to primary care as a rich source of learning opportunities, and of course primary care is the obvious location to teach GP registrars. It is becoming hard to avoid medical students and GP registrars in general practices. This is also not a role that most medical graduates are trained for.
- Teamwork skills. General practice is now recognised as being most effective when medical practitioners, nurses, physiotherapists, receptionists, etc. (in fact the whole healthcare team) work together. Each team member should understand team processes and be prepared to assume part of the responsibility for the outcomes of team effort. Teamwork is difficult to teach except through role-modelling. This teamwork concept is most advanced in the UK healthcare system, where practice nurses play a more independent role, and team meetings take place more often, incorporating the perspectives of several different health professions into patient care.

This role description could be awesome and overwhelming. It is important to recognise that the traditional model of general practice, in which the family GP personally provided comprehensive 24-hour care for a lifetime, is disappearing. General practice now offers a range of practice styles and special interests. The above principles can be provided within a structure that allows GPs to collaborate with nurses and other community workers on the provision of after-hours care and on illness prevention and health promotion. This collaboration requires teamwork skills that many individualistic GPs have not had in the past. In essence, we need GPs who will 'work smarter', not harder. We should not be trying to train 'superdocs', but rather doctors who will perform well their role within the healthcare system.

More recent changes are contributing to an even more different future. Recent graduates are less likely to stay in one practice location for their whole career, and also less likely to stay in the same branch of the profession for long. Instead, people now change careers through re-skilling, either within or outside of medicine and the medical profession. The 'skills escalator' concept is becoming a reality. Further changes are being forced by workforce issues. As other specialties narrow and become more technology based, primary care is assuming some of the roles of the former generalist specialists, and practice nurses and psychologists are assuming some of the former general practice medical roles – the 'job substitution' concept.

Other authors have encapsulated the conceptual basis of general practice very well. These are listed under 'Further Reading' below.

Characteristics of a good general practitioner

Good GPs possess many attributes, although few (if any) individuals possess all desirable attributes. Just as general practice is a diverse discipline, GPs come in many varieties and flavours. Perhaps the most important attributes are as follows:

- sound working knowledge of a wide range of health and disease processes
- sound clinical skills that enable a wide range of problems to be managed
- communication skills that make them approachable and understanding
- understanding of their role in the healthcare system
- understanding of population health principles, even though the focus of their routine work is the care of individuals
- ability to help patients learn about their health
- appropriate ethical and professional behaviour
- organisational and time management skills
- ability to reflect on practice, thus facilitating continuing professional development
- a happy balance of professional and personal lives.

After reading this feelings of inadequacy might arise! However, even if we do not feel as perfect as this may sound, these are the kinds of attributes that clinical supervisors should be trying to demonstrate to learners.

The nature of teaching and learning in general practice

Learning, in the context of medical education, is more than the acquisition of knowledge, skills and attitudes. A complete definition must include the concepts of *meaning* and *application*. Successful learning requires information to be relevant to practice and to be incorporated into practice. This is a little different to some definitions of learning and might upset purists. What is wrong, one might ask, with simply acquiring new information? New information can give the appearance of being erudite and is useful in a trivia quiz. However, there is a difference between knowing and doing, and the focus of learning in medicine is to produce a set of informed behaviours. Hence, the focus of medical education is maintaining or improving performance in practice in order to provide the highest quality healthcare for the community.

Reflect for a moment on your own experiences as a learner. Who were the most effective teachers in your life? What did they teach you? What do you remember most about what they taught? What were their most effective teaching strategies? Think about the worst teachers you have had. What did they do that really bothered you? What were their least effective teaching strategies?

Many of the most positive experiences will have involved learning from people who were not necessarily experts in the discipline. It can be an error to assume that only senior clinicians can be effective teachers. Increasingly, the valuable role that more junior clinicians can play is being recognised. The most effective teachers are often only two or three years ahead of learners on the career progress scale. For example, senior students can learn a lot from registrars, who have a more recent experience of the curriculum and can often make it more accessible to those not far behind: after all, this is the way most junior hospital doctors learn. Similarly, junior medical students can learn a lot from senior medical students. Further, registrars can learn a lot from GPs who have only recently completed training and achieved recognition as a GP. One positive outcome of involving senior students and registrars in teaching is that it helps to train and to role-model the next generation of teaching clinicians. Teaching is an implicit part of the role of medical practitioners, yet preparation for this role is sadly lacking. Ideally, teacher training should be a part of mainstream medical education for all students and registrars.

Teaching is really about facilitation of learning. It is about inspiring and guiding learners to pursue the knowledge, skills and understanding that will make them better clinicians. It is difficult to stop learners learning, although poor teaching practices can impede or misdirect learning. It is also difficult to define teaching, as there are many different models. This is discussed further in Chapter 4.

The nature of practice attachments

A practice attachment could be defined broadly as a period of 'real practice' learning, when the curriculum might comprise aspects of whatever the supervising clinician is doing. Attachments vary in their duration, intensity, location and timing according to their purpose within a training programme. Medical school attachments tend to be shorter than postgraduate attachments and are more often less than full-time. A newer form of attachment is the *longitudinal* general practice attachment, where medical students may be attached for only part of each week, but perhaps for a whole academic year. This allows for better integration of primary and secondary care experiences. Because practices are different from each other, each attachment tends to offer a somewhat individual experience, so learners might benefit from having a range of practices from which to choose an experience that is more relevant to their needs. Further, learners might learn more if they spent time in more than one practice.

Learners come to practice attachments at a particular point in their learning pathway. Sometimes this is quite early when the purpose is to provide general exposure to patients in a primary healthcare setting. Alternatively, it could be for communication skills training or, for more advanced learners, acquisition of guided but fairly autonomous experience. The point is that practice attachments are simply part of an overall curriculum plan that is required by the relevant educational organisation. It is important for clinical supervisors to know exactly what learners are supposed to be gaining from the attachment, and how this fits in with the broader curriculum. These issues are discussed in later chapters.

The nature of practice attachments is broadening as educational organisations shift the emphasis of their teaching and learning away from in-patient hospital facilities towards the community. This shift is occurring because in-patient care is now reserved for a restricted range of patients and conditions. The cost of in-patient care means that admissions are now brief, allowing for intensive investigation and management of relatively complex clinical conditions. An increasing proportion of the clinical case-mix of hospitals is now short-stay (same day admissions) for an increasing range of investigations and procedures. The cost of in-patient care is so high that ambulatory care is becoming increasingly sophisticated, with early discharge, home IV and other community-based programmes that keep people out of hospital.

Hence general practice is being seen as an ideal place for medical students to learn things that were once only available in hospitals, including basic clinical skills. Here the focus is less on the nature of general practice and more on opportunities to learn from patients who are more accessible than hospital in-patients. As medical education expands this is now often done with groups of students on short-term attachments, rather than the traditional one-to-one attachment. This requires a different approach to one-to-one supervision, so a later chapter deals with small group practice-based teaching.

Primary care and medical education

General practice has also changed from the traditional, individual doctor-oriented model to one where GPs more often work in group practices that include several GPs, practice nurses and potentially a wide range of other health professionals. Patients are more likely to regards the *practice* as the constant, and be prepared to consult the nurse where that is more appropriate or easier. Practice nurses will make an assessment that may result in them managing the encounter or, where necessary, triaging and referring the patient to one of the GPs. The GPs within the practice work together, sharing patients and perhaps each providing particular services that indicate a degree of specialisation or special interest. Examples include sports medicine and women's health. Further, special clinics are often provided to manage patients with hypertension, diabetes, obesity or other chronic or complex problems. Practices do not really compete with each other, but collaborate through their local primary care trust to provide services to their respective practice populations. Although patients can change practices quite easily, this is still a relatively infrequent event. Trusts 'purchase' services from practices, and provide incentives for achieving targets for immunisation and other health prevention programmes, ensure patient access to a wide range of primary healthcare providers through general practices, but including home visits, and coordinate primary care and hospital services. Practice cooperatives increasingly provide regional after-hours care, often using practice nurses as for initial assessment and triage. GPs are often the managers of this broader, multi-professional approach (that is changing), but they are not the only source of information, opinion and management. This model has broken down some of the cross-sectoral barriers in the healthcare system and has almost certainly improved coordination of healthcare.

It is important that the whole range of primary care practice activity is made available to learners, who can benefit from observing and helping to assess patients as they go through this more integrated primary care system. Registrars should be able to become involved as much as the practice principals, once they are comfortable with the process and know how to access advice. Medical students will play a more observational role, but can learn a lot from the other health professionals. Ideally, their supervisors should role-model positive team involvement and the patients should have demonstrably improved outcomes. More senior students can also be allocated tasks that contribute to the team assessment. One example is that a student could be asked to review the medications taken by a patient with multiple problems, and present this for discussion at a team meeting.

Fitting teaching in: time management

One of the essential skills of efficient GPs is time management. Busy clinicians must fit in the demands of patients, practice management, self-management and personal issues. This is not easy and we should not be surprised that few do it well. The addition of a teaching commitment, whatever the level of enthusiasm, can add to the chaos and make life even more difficult. Without adequate time management, either the clinical care, teaching or personal life can suffer. The result will be a poor learning experience and frustration for the supervisor.

The secret to achieving a calm balance between potentially conflicting roles is in scheduling. Just as appointments for patients spread the clinical workload over a manageable time-frame, making appointments for teaching time ensures that teaching occurs in a stress-free environment. Walk-in clinics are generally less useful for teaching medical students, as controlling the workload is difficult, unless simply observing the more acute nature of the work is regarded as a useful opportunity (only once!). Times for contact with learners should be scheduled and protected. When the learner is sitting in with the general practitioner, fewer consultations should be booked so that there is time for adequate discussion of each case. Australian research evidence suggests that good teaching slows doctors down by 25–30%. Clearly, the key to successful clinical teaching is prior planning.

Scheduling time for teaching is easier in a group practice, as other practice members can absorb the extra workload while one devotes time to teach. This task is more difficult for practices in areas of greater healthcare need, such as rural and deprived urban communities. These GPs are likely to be busier, caring for populations with a relatively heavy patient morbidity and after-hours load. More remote practices are also more likely to be sole practices. One could ask if sole-practitioner practices should ever be accredited teaching practices, as there is less flexibility. However, current workforce data indicate that learners need to encounter successful rural practice role models, so rural supervisors must adapt their teaching practices to allow them to meet both clinical and educational roles.

Other strategies can be influenced at the practice level through efficient use of time and learning strategies. Depending on the level of the learner (i.e. junior medical student through to advanced GP registrar), supervisors do not have to be present for all learning activities. Some tips for efficient use of time for teaching are listed in Box 1.1. Supervisors should identify a range of activities that learners could usefully do in the practice, some of which rely on other staff members. These should reflect the learning objectives of the attachment. For example, medical students could: sit in with all practice doctors, including GP registrars; see patients independently; observe receptionist and nursing staff; retrieve and file patient records; visit nearby pharmacists, physiotherapists, etc.; and spend time reading journals and books. In fact, many students find prolonged sitting in boring, and supervisors get behind with their other work. Thoughtful scheduling of a range of relevant activities frees the supervisor to get on with other priorities. At the level of GP registrars, a similar range of activities might be useful, but the primary purpose of the attachment is to allow the learner to gain experience from as many patient encounters as is reasonable. This does not mean that GP registrars should be under pressure to see more patients than they can cope with. There should be time for reflection and discussion of each case.

Box 1.1 Menu of teaching and learning activities that can improve efficiency of practice-based teaching

- Sitting in with all practice partners
- Sitting in with learners of a higher level, e.g. medical student with GP registrar
- Working in the reception area
- Working with the practice nurse
- Working with the community pharmacist and other health professionals
- Personal reflection and study time
- Use travel time and social events
- Time allowed in lieu of after-hours work

Supervisors should also use non-patient contact time efficiently. For example, important issues can be discussed during a drive to a home or nursing-home visit. Similarly, coffee and meal breaks are opportunities for discussion of the day's cases. After-hours contact should also be made, for both social and work reasons. Learners should gain an appreciation of how GPs balance personal and professional demands, and hosting them for a meal will help show this. Sadly, some students are shown rather poorly balanced lives, which they remember, so supervisors must be careful to attend to some self-care before exposing the balance in their personal lives. Learners at all levels could focus more on after-hours presentations, using in-hours time to seek resources and reflect. This offers some interesting presentations and also exposes learners to an important part of general practice. Often there is more time for discussion of cases and there should be opportunities for follow-up within the next few days.

Allocation of time for learners to undertake self-directed study is an excellent idea. Learners appreciate time to ensure that they have covered the learning objectives of the attachment and may want to do this in their own way. Learning can be built around cases seen earlier, such that the learner follows a patient through a hospital admission and reads the relevant literature, then reports back on progress and future management options. This requires some resources, such as access to a range of books, journals and electronic databases. All teaching practices should have a range of key textbooks, relevant journals, and computers with, ideally, broadband access to the web, including access to the Royal College of General Practitioners (RCGP) Resource. The bottom line is that clinical supervisors agree to do a certain amount of educational work. They should either meet, or reconsider, this commitment. Doing the job poorly leaves the learner, supervisor and educational organisation unhappy. The importance of careful planning will be seen again in later chapters.

Fitting teaching in: space considerations

As practices become more efficient businesses it has also become clear that teaching requires additional space and resources. Clearly registrars need their own consulting room, clinical equipment, computer, access to the information technology (IT) system, and access to nurse and receptionist support. However, medical students also need to learn by doing, albeit with closer supervision, and little is achieved if students simply sit on a chair tucked into a corner for more than just the introductory sessions.

Hence the modern teaching practice now requires a room, a computer, clinical equipment, access to the IT system and access to practice staff for medical students, particularly the more senior students. This means that they can get more out of patient interactions by becoming a junior member of the medical team, taking histories and examining patients before presenting them to their supervisors. Similar facilities are also needed for more junior students, although they can be shared by a small group of students.

Being a teaching practice is an additional professional role that is often not funded clearly through traditional health service budgets. Sadly, it is not always thought of in education budgets either, although more recently constructed practice facilities will almost certainly include teaching space and facilities if the practice is an accredited teaching practice.

The rewards of the teaching role

Why should clinicians take on a teaching role? The real rewards are usually quite intrinsic and personal. Some feel like variety after years of continuous, full-time clinical work. Clinical teachers often find that having learners is the best form of continuing medical education (CME), as students and GP registrars constantly challenge their knowledge and reasoning. The teaching role also opens up new networks of friends and colleagues with similar interests. Most enjoy the role. A few are interested in exploring a more academic career.

One of the relative advantages of the UK healthcare system is that there are also genuine extrinsic rewards for being a recognised trainer, particularly in the vocational training scheme. Registrars come with a full salary, and so can actually relieve principals of patient contact time, freeing them for teaching. Teaching time is protected and paid for within the practice, and practice staffing and organisation are designed to support the teaching role. Teacher training is provided and funded, including the GP salary for attendance time. There is a strong mutual support organisation for GP trainers, with its own journal (*Education for Primary Care*). This somewhat idyllic description is not always present and can vary from region to region, but in comparison with teaching practices in Australia and New Zealand, the picture is rosy.

In undergraduate teaching, the resources are often less generous and can vary more between regions and medical schools. Teaching time is still paid for, academic titles can be conferred, access to research support and libraries is available, and teacher training is supported. However, GPs teaching in medical schools are not usually the managers or primary educators of their learners, and their status within medical schools can be lower. While many GP trainers are involved in both undergraduate and vocational training levels, there is some differentiation of interest and organisational influence.

The complications of a teaching role

Learning is about personal growth. When teaching is relatively well supported, individual practitioners can choose whether or not to change the balance in their professional lives by replacing some clinical interest with an educational interest. We learn about many things, as our lives are multifaceted. In the professional sense, we often concentrate a lot of time and resources into maintaining currency with clinical practice, as that is our acknowledged role in society. Those of us who are involved in teaching also need to learn how to do that, and then to maintain those skills, as we have an obligation to nurture those who will ultimately replace us. This of course complicates continuing professional development, as practice supervisors should choose to attend regular educational, as well as clinical, sessions. The answer lies in *balance.*

Self-care

One thing that clinical supervisors should not do is to simply add teaching responsibilities to otherwise hectic lives. That way lies further complications and time pressures that will ultimately limit the enjoyment of teaching and also impair its quality. The teaching role requires freedom from other commitments, although the financial constraints are acknowledged. Further, taking on a teaching load for the whole year might not be advisable, unless clinical and administrative workloads can be arranged to support that. It is a good idea to host learners intermittently, so that supervisors can have a rest from their teaching role and can arrange release from some other duties for the times that they do host learners. All supervisors, particularly those who are more popular, should be prepared to say 'no' to an educational organisation if an attachment cannot be supported appropriately.

Contemporary issues in medical education

One of the challenges facing the entire medical profession at the moment is the push to reform the rather long and inflexible medical training programmes. After five, six or seven years to attain a basic medical degree, graduates undertake one to three years (often more) of general hospital training, followed by four to seven years of specialty training. There is little recognition of prior learning (RPL), so individuals who change training programmes usually have to start again. Further, most training programmes do not have common, recognised experiences where graduates could start and then narrow training after a year or two. Still further, the 'pure' apprenticeship model is no longer regarded as sufficient, as it is probably too reliant on time and passive experience. The near future may well see compression of total training programme time, intensive modules that enhance experience, greater commonality and cross-recognition of general experience, and increased recognition of prior learning. The result, at least in theory, may be a more flexible medical workforce that can adapt to community healthcare needs.

Another challenge is how to address the safety and quality concerns of funders, regulators and patients. While the profession accepts that there may be an unavoidable error rate in medical decision making, many stakeholders are now aware that this is almost certainly too high. Errors may be due to poor performance by individuals, but are increasingly recognised as being 'system' issues, many of which are potentially avoidable. Error rates are difficult to measure, but iatrogenesis is a common cause of documented morbidity and mortality in hospital settings in both Australia and North America (Brennan *et al.*, 1991; Wilson *et al.*, 1999), and the situation may be similar in primary care. The Bristol and Shipman cases in the UK have focused attention on clinical governance, or the system-wide approach to shared responsibility for prevention and management of safety and quality concerns. Skirting the debate for now, the message for educators is that education programmes, their curricula, assessment and evaluation, will from now on have to address the safety and quality of the practice agenda.

Summary

Clinical supervision is a challenging, yet rewarding, professional role. This chapter acts as an introduction to a practical book that will assist readers to travel along an enlightening professional development journey that should result in a more satisfying career as an experienced clinician and wise clinical supervisor, based on a sound knowledge and understanding of educational principles. Subsequent chapters present some educational concepts and theory and many practical examples of how to help learners gain the most from an attachment in clinical practice.

Further reading

McWhinney IR (1997) *A Textbook of Family Medicine* (2e). Oxford: Oxford University Press.
  This provides an overview of the nature of general/family practice. Often recommended as a text in medical schools, it is well worth reading and revising at any stage of career development. McWhinney is particularly strong on the conceptual basis of the discipline.
Jones R, Britten N, Culpepper L *et al.* (eds) (2004) *Oxford Textbook of Primary Medical Care.* Oxford: Oxford University Press.
  Award-winning, very comprehensive international textbook on primary medical care with contributions from many leading academics around the world. This transplants quite well into most national systems as there are chapters on the differences and similarities for each nation, compared with the more generic materials. It is risky suggesting that readers go through this huge, two-volume set, but it really does contain almost everything one might want to know about the discipline of general practice in its wider primary care professional context.

Chapter 2

What can general practice teach?

> To live for a while close to great minds is the best kind of education.
> John Buchan

General practice attachments are essential sites of general practice learning, but are not the only sites. Indeed, there are some things that learners can learn more effectively in hospitals and in tutorials or other formal sessions, just as some things can be learned only in general practice attachments. The range of clinical topics that can be covered in primary care depends primarily on the range of patients encountered, and to a lesser extent on the breadth and depth of expertise of the supervising health professionals. Specific expertise is not always essential: for example, a general practitioner may not be able to discuss the detailed clinical pathology of skin lesions, but will be able to provide learners with access to several patients with skin lesions, thereby giving meaning to what has been learned from a dermatologist. It is these learning opportunities that allow learners to integrate theory and practice in a way that strengthens both. This chapter explores what is best learned in general practice, and how this relates to a curriculum that guides learning throughout an entire training programme.

The relevance of a curriculum

Supervisors may be asked to supervise students and/or registrars who must follow different curricula. For example, there are several medical schools within close proximity in several UK cities, and several regional training programmes. Diversity is now valued in medical education, so each medical school will work towards common learning outcomes for their degrees, but may well try to add different 'flavours' or characteristics to their graduates. For example, medical schools may strive to produce the next generation of academic leaders at the forefront of technology, or they may adopt a socially accountable approach to producing graduates that meet regional needs. These may of course not be incompatible goals! Similarly, regional vocational training providers will work towards having graduates meeting Joint Committee on Postgraduate Training for General Practice (JCPTGP) objectives, but in different ways. These differences may simply require learners to do similar things in a different sequence or a different context, but it is worthwhile knowing a little about curriculum development in order to understand the role of practice-based teaching.

A curriculum is a statement of what is to be learned. It is similar to a road map, in that it indicates a destination, directions for getting there and points along the way for rest, refuelling and reflection on how the journey has gone. The road map analogy is particularly appropriate for general practice attachments, because there is often more than one way to reach the destination. The precise path chosen should depend on the negotiations between supervisor and learner.

All training programmes should have some form of documented curriculum, ideally developed with the assistance of a range of stakeholders and interest groups, and therefore reflecting reasonable consensus on what the graduate of the training programme should know and do. Curriculum documents vary considerably in their content, but should contain an overall goal or aim that describes the desired outcome, a set of measurable educational objectives and a description of the entire curriculum. Ideally, the educational processes to be employed throughout the entire course, at least in broad terms, are included. This chapter dips into some educational theory so that supervisors can better understand the origin of the tasks they are given by the educational organisation.

Curriculum structure

The structure and level of detail in curricula vary considerably. Curricula should have an overall goal or mission and a list of learning objectives, ideally based on a nationally (soon perhaps internationally) agreed list of desirable attributes of 'good' medical practitioners. These lists are usually produced by state or national medical councils, and include attributes in addition to the traditional knowledge and skills, such as issues relevant to personal and professional behaviour. Further, in many nations doctors are expected to be collaborators/team players, communicators, advocates and scholars. Examples of some of these are listed under 'Further Reading' below. Learning objectives should be accompanied by a detailed description of how they can be achieved, and they should be measurable.

The current approach is to express curriculum content in terms of 'domains' of competence, or conceptual themes of ideas and attributes required by competent professionals, with other information that guides educational development, such as age groups, presenting complaints or systems. Actual data on what problems present to general practitioners is available, so this approach is evidence-based. The International Classification of Primary Care (ICPC) is a useful means of defining clinical content for primary care, as this describes problems rather than diagnoses. Domain titles often use terms that describe knowledge, skills and attitudes under titles such as 'applied clinical knowledge', 'clinical and communication skills' and 'ethical, personal and professional behaviour'. Despite the different names, domains often overlap to some extent in terms of their content. The result is a 'universe' of competence, containing a number of 'components of competence', that in combination define a competent practitioner. This information is often summarised in a curriculum blueprint, a very basic example of which is provided in Table 2.1. Each box represents a component of competence that reflects a content area under ICPC headings (column) and domain of competence (row). In this example, only a single topic is provided for each content area, although clearly there are many that would be included in a genuine blueprint. Some domain-specific issues, such as writing certificates, are relevant for more than the specified content topic, and would not necessarily need to be repeated for all conditions. There would also normally be many more columns, reflecting a complete classification of primary care presentations.

Table 2.1 An example of a basic curriculum blueprint

	Content area (International Classification of Primary Care)				
Domains	Respiratory	Cardio-vascular	Neurology	Uncertain	Musculo-skeletal
Knowledge	Asthma symptoms	Causes of hypertension	Causes of headache	Acute fevers in children	Causes of low back pain
Clinical skills	Explaining management plan	Optic fundi examination	Central nervous system examination	Recognising severe illness	Back examination skills
Doctor and community	Barriers to early presentation	Regular screening of blood pressure of practice patients	Prevalence of migraine	Vaccination schedules	Occupational health and safety awareness
Ethical and professional	Provision of after-hours support	When to refer	Avoidance of inappropriate narcotic use	Arrangements for review	Writing certificates

Sometimes blueprints are complex, three-dimensional figures, as age and gender of patients might be relevant to all issues defined by presenting complaint and domain. This does not matter, so long as there is broad agreement on its meaning by relevant stakeholders. A blueprint is more a conceptual framework than a precise definition, although it should 'map' curriculum content and the relationship of components to each other, as a guide to learners. In theory, learners should know something in each of the blueprint squares. Course organisers can look at the whole blueprint and determine what should be taught by lectures, tutorials, workshops and practice-based supervision. Clinical supervisors and learners can also inspect these documents and understand the relevance of their practice experiences to the broader picture. A blueprint is also essential to rational assessment, as it can also guide test item selection, thus ensuring that learners are assessed on what they should learn. More of the assessment role of blueprinting is presented in Chapter 3.

A curriculum may be linear, in that learners progress together at the same rate and in the same sequence, or it may be modular, in that discrete portions of the curriculum may be taken in varied sequences. The latter is the more common approach taken in higher education, as it allows the more self-directed approach that is preferred by adult learners. One topical method of defining a curriculum for such a broad discipline as general practice is the 'core plus options' model (Harden and Davis, 1995). Many GPs have particular interests and skills that are not required by all GPs, but all will need to follow a similar curriculum pathway to ensure that 'core' issues are covered. Hence a number of modules are mandatory for all learners, while other modules are offered for those choosing to gain particular knowledge and skills outside the core. The process of determining what is core and what is optional is difficult. Just what learners are required to cover during the practice attachment should be made clear by the relevant educational organisation.

The relationship between the actual and potential curriculum

Curriculum blueprints often have the effect of making curricula appear to be quite compact, with components of competency appearing to have precise relationships with each other. This is not often the way it is, but the simpler representation is a useful way of organising learning. Another way of viewing a curriculum is to consider its relationship to curricula for other disciplines. Particularly in primary care professions, a diverse range of presentations may confront practitioners. Hence the potential curriculum for a GP is vast – including parts of all other disciplines – and is too large to cover formally during a defined training period. Therefore, curriculum designers should identify only the domain content that should be covered by all learners (the core/options approach), and then consider how this content relates to other medical disciplines. This concept is depicted in Figure 2.1, which shows that a general practice curriculum is within the 'universe' of medical curriculum issues, but is not necessarily a neat segment that is separated from the content of other medical disciplines.

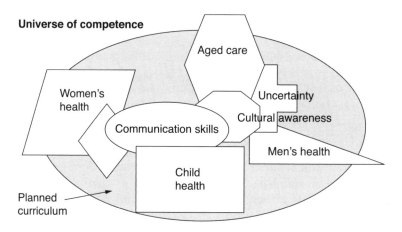

Figure 2.1 The relationship between the actual and the potential curriculum.

The figure might make the choices appear to be haphazard, but they are not, as they should reflect careful consideration of the roles and responsibilities of GPs within the broader healthcare system. Curriculum topics, listed here as women's health, child health, communication skills, etc. (rather than systems, as in Table 2.1), are likely to overlap. Further, not all of the curriculum will fit neatly into domains. There might be gaps (the shaded areas) that should still be learned, not necessarily in precise modules, but rather through self-study or experience. Precise content is likely to vary between healthcare systems.

Different kinds of curricula

So far the discussion has focused on the construction of a formal curriculum – the 'planned' curriculum. However, even if this is done well, it may not be the curriculum that learners receive. There are two other forms of curriculum that supervisors should be aware of, as they have the power either to follow the curriculum provided by the educational organisation, or to guide learning in a different direction.

The first is the 'taught' curriculum, or what the learners actually experience. Formal curricula are often not delivered as they are planned, because either the curriculum cannot be delivered as planned, the teachers do not deliver it as planned, or the learners are subjected to additional experiences that were not planned. This often relates to poor curriculum development or lack of participation of teachers in the development process. An example might be a curriculum that places strong emphasis on the teaching and learning of ethical and professional behaviours, but then fails to place the same emphasis on the implementation of the curriculum. Poorly selected practice-based teachers might not role-model the desired behaviours or might even demonstrate poor ethical and professional behaviours.

The second is the 'assessed curriculum'. This reflects the all too frequent mismatch between the formal curriculum and what is assessed. An example might be a curriculum that places emphasis on ethical and professional behaviours, role-models these well in clinical practice attachments, but then does not assess these attributes. Learners are human and will direct their learning to where there is a perceived reward; if assessment does not reinforce the message that ethical and professional behaviours are essential to competent practice, then learners will concentrate on the knowledge and skills that are assessed. In essence, the assessment 'tail' wags the curriculum 'dog'.

Ideally, there is congruence between the planned curriculum, how it is delivered and how learners are assessed. This is represented conceptually in Figure 2.2. The weaker the level of congruence, the greater the degree of what is called the 'hidden curriculum', which includes elements of the planned, taught and assessed curricula. However, while it may not be the intended learning outcome, this is what learners really learn. A hidden curriculum has the potential to impede progress towards achievement of desired learning objectives. It is best avoided by appropriate curriculum development, such that there is congruence between what stakeholders desire to be the outcome, the process for implementing the curriculum and the assessment practices. Clinical supervisors have an important role in ensuring that formal curricula are both deliverable and delivered as intended, as the academics who develop curricula may not appreciate the practical issues of teaching and learning in community settings.

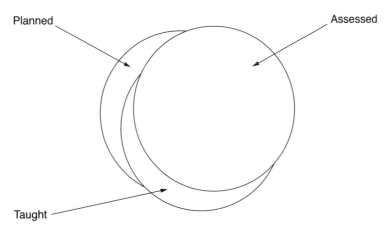

Figure 2.2 Clashing curricula: the importance of congruence in curriculum design, implementation and assessment.

The curriculum for a practice attachment

This manual does not attempt to provide a curriculum for practice attachment, for two reasons. The first is that the content will span several issues that are better dealt with elsewhere. Clinical content is not presented, as this manual is more about concepts and the process of practice-based teaching. A list of additional resources, where relevant, is provided under 'Further Reading' at the end of each chapter. These resources include books, journals and internet websites. The second reason is that the curriculum will vary according to the nature of the educational organisation, the context of the practice and the level of the learner. Different organisations will expect practice-based teaching to fit into their overall curricula in a particular way, although the strengths of practice-based teaching mean that there will be some similarity, whatever the organisation.

Strengths of practice-based teaching

The power of clinical supervision lies in the ability of learners to gain experience of healthcare and to model their professional behaviour on that of their supervisors. The emphasis will be on seeing, doing and receiving feedback, as practice attachments are where learners will see a wide range of ordinary patients with common problems. Practice-based teaching is not so much about acquiring knowledge, but working out how to apply that knowledge in a practical way. Specific learning objectives for practice attachments might include:

- Broad understanding of general practice and community-based care. This is appropriate for medical students and other early learners.
- Contextual issues. A good example is rural healthcare, which is demonstrated better in a rural setting than in an urban lecture (*see* Chapter 3).
- Communication skills. Learners at all levels benefit from talking with patients about their problems, although skills chosen will depend on the level of the learner.
- Clinical skills. Medical students benefit from practising basic skills such as taking blood pressures, listening to chests, examining joints, etc. and should have several opportunities to do this with patients with both normal and abnormal signs. GP registrars will want to learn more advanced procedures.
- Practical procedures. Medical students will need practice at giving injections, ear syringing, suturing, urine dipstick testing, pinprick blood sugar levels, etc. GP registrars will need more advanced skills such as Pap smears, removing skin lesions, applying plaster casts, etc. The precise nature of the experience depends on the workload and the setting.
- The general practice clinical method. GPs work differently from other specialists, in that they deal with a wide range of problems quite quickly. They deal with low prior probabilities of serious illness, yet must be able to detect when more thorough investigation is required. They have now also adopted a major role in illness prevention. Medical students will need to be aware of these differences, but GP registrars will need to gain considerable practice of the method. More on this later.
- Ethical and professional behaviours. Many of these are attitudinal, and are difficult to 'teach'. They are best learned in clinical practice rather than in lectures through observing doctors behaving ethically and professionally in

many clinical scenarios. Ethical and professional issues are often at the root of performance problems referred to regulatory authorities, so are now being taken more seriously.

- Teamwork skills. GPs are part of a healthcare team and should be able to demonstrate their role in what is a complex, multi-professional environment. They must be able to work with each other, with other health professionals and with regulatory authorities.
- Time management skills. We are often not as good at time management as we think! The best way to 'teach' this is to demonstrate a sound approach to scheduling clinical, practice management, educational and personal roles.

Problem solving in general practice

The general practice clinical method is really a rapid problem-solving approach that can deal efficiently with a variety of presenting complaints. We pride ourselves on this ability and watch in bemusement as our learners struggle to keep pace. There is a temptation to try to teach this skill by explaining what is going through our minds as we proceed through the consultation. However, before trying, clinical supervisors should understand how clinicians solve problems.

There are two ways in which doctors solve clinical problems. The first way is that we gather information, piece it together to form a hypothesis (or diagnosis) and then try to find information which confirms or refutes that hypothesis. This is called the hypothetico-deductive model of clinical reasoning. It is particularly useful for new, unusual or complex presentations. It can be slow, but is thorough. Not surprisingly, this is the way that learners start out in practice.

However, it is not the way that experienced clinicians function most of the time. With experience, most presentations 'have been seen before'. Particularly when the doctor knows the patient, the patient's presenting complaint often fast-tracks thought processes to the point where a strong diagnostic impression is already present based on what might be called 'elaborated knowledge'. Fewer questions need to be asked to confirm this impression, so the whole process is over rapidly. This is called 'pattern matching'.

The two forms of problem solving are represented in Figure 2.3 as jigsaw puzzles. Figure 2.3a is the hypothetico-deductive model, where the picture is complex and the jigsaw has a large number of smaller pieces. In order to guess what the picture is, the problem-solver needs to acquire many, possibly most, of the pieces placed strategically around the jigsaw. Skill is required to seek the strategically relevant information. Figure 2.3b is 'pattern matching', where the picture appears to be simpler and the jigsaw has fewer, larger pieces. The number of pieces required to solve the problem is small. Sometimes a single piece suffices, the so-called 'spot diagnosis'. This is not a derogatory concept, but rather the way experienced GPs work much of the time.

What is the difference between more complex problems such as those in Figure 2.3a and simpler problems such as those in Figure 2.3b? Usually, the answer is experience. Problems that challenge learners might appear simple to an experienced clinician who has seen similar presentations many times before. Referring back to Figure 2.3b, those who spend a lot of time in airports will recognise that the scene depicted is an airport lounge. People without that prior experience might struggle with only a single puzzle piece provided. (See p. 118 for full images.)

(a) Hypothetico-deductive

(b) Pattern matching

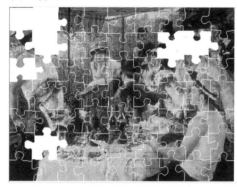 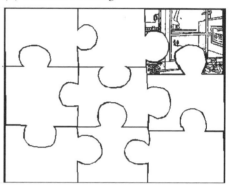

Figure 2.3 The hypothetico-deductive and pattern matching models.

The point is that pattern matching cannot be taught, but it can be learned. The most effective way of learning clinical problem solving is to encounter large numbers of clinical presentations. Hence an important role of clinical supervisors is to ensure that their learners gain experience of several examples in each of a wide range of patient presentations, and to discuss with them the variations that help include or exclude possible diagnoses. In time, jigsaw puzzle pieces become larger and the picture appears simpler. The implications for practice-based teaching are that the experience of learners needs to be monitored to ensure a broad experience of clinical medicine. It is insufficient to assume that a suitable range of presentations will appear, so 'arranging' appropriate consultations is often required. Secondly, learners should be confronted by more complex or unusual presentations that stimulate practice of the hypothetico-deductive method, which all practitioners must fall back on when confronted by unusual presentations that do not fit prior experience. However, this is not an argument for learners to be pressured to see too many patients – there must be a balance between seeing/doing and reflecting/discussing in order to reinforce learning.

Helping learners at different career levels

Practice-based teaching can be applied to learners at different levels and with different expectations. These include secondary school students on work experience, medical students at any stage of the course, and GP registrars in basic, advanced or mentor terms. More recently, the increasingly globalised medical workforce situation has seen a new level of learner emerge: international medical graduates, with varying levels and kinds of experiences, who require at least a period of supervision until they adapt to the local healthcare system, but also possibly substantial retraining, rather like (yet still different from) GP registrars. The needs of individuals at each level are different, so practice-based teaching methods must be tailored to the needs of both the particular group and the individual. This tailoring is one of the skills that clinical supervisors need to acquire, and is presented in more detail in Chapter 4.

Broadly speaking, there is a spectrum of issues and topics that are relevant to learners at, and within, each level. This is summarised in Table 2.2, overleaf. This is purely indicative, as all issues are relevant to some extent at both medical school and postgraduate levels, but differences in emphasis are needed at different levels. Early emphasis is on observing, later emphasis is on doing. Junior medical students require exposure to general practice and community care concepts, communication skills practice and some basic clinical skills such as simple clinical examination techniques. Senior medical students need these, plus experience of specific clinical topics (e.g. treating URTIs) and opportunities to practise interviewing skills and some practical procedures. At the postgraduate level, basic-term registrars need time to come to grips with the differences between hospital and community care, the mechanics of private practice prescribing and referrals, and solving problems within a restricted time period. More advanced registrars need to grapple with more complex clinical management issues, and should learn about practice management, as soon they might be responsible for this. Issues such as communication skills, clinical skills and practical procedures are relevant at all levels, but the precise nature of skills will change from simpler to more advanced. For example, a year one medical student might need practise at taking blood pressures, whereas advanced GP registrars might need to learn how to fit an intrauterine device or do simple rotational flaps. Ethical and professional behaviours should be role-modelled in all settings, but with more advanced learners opportunities should be taken to discuss ethical issues as they arise. More advanced learners also need to learn how to cope with uncertainty.

Several medical schools are adopting graduate entry and problem-based learning courses, so the characteristics of medical students and roles of practice attachments might vary between universities. GPs taking students from these new courses might wonder whether the students are so different that a different educational approach is required during practice attachments. The obvious differences between students at 'traditional' (undergraduate) and graduate courses are summarised in Table 2.3, overleaf. Graduate course students all have a prior university degree. In theory, they are often a little older, their backgrounds more diverse, their motivation to study medicine higher and their independent learning skills better than students in non-graduate entry courses.

Table 2.2 Relevance of some curriculum issues according to the level of the learner

Issue	Junior medical student	Senior medical student	Less advanced GP registrar	More advanced GP registrar
Exposure to GP	+++	++	+	−
Healthcare system	+	++	+++	−
Communication	+++	+++	++	+
Consulting skills	+	++	+++	+++
Examination skills	++	+	+	−
Procedural skills	+	+	+++	++
Clinical topics	++	++	+++	++
Ethics	+	+	++	+++
Uncertainty	+	+	+++	++
Self-care	−	+	++	+++
Practice management	−	−	+	+++

It is gradually becoming apparent that the differences may not be as clear-cut as originally thought. One difference that has emerged is that older students are more likely to have partners with careers, children and jobs to meet financial obligations, and so have to balance study and personal lives more than younger students. Relocation for longer rural placements is more difficult at both undergraduate and vocational training levels; by the time the latter happens, older students are more likely to have partners entrenched in careers and school-age children.

Medical student cohorts have always included some older, more independent students. Further, most medical schools use interviews as part of their selection processes, aiming to select students with strong interpersonal skills and the potential for more independent learning. The impression is that graduate entry course students may be more accustomed to a more independent, resource-based learning approach, but it is not clear how much of this is due to the nature of the curriculum, rather than the attributes of students.

Table 2.3 Attributes of graduate entry and undergraduate entry medical students

Graduate entry programme	Undergraduate entry programme
All have prior degrees	A minority have prior degrees
More have had prior careers	Fewer have had prior careers
More older students	Fewer older students
More used to resource-based learning	More used to didactic teaching
More assertive about needs	More accepting of what is offered
More mature decision and motivation to study medicine	Decision to study medicine made at a younger age

Hence, regardless of the selection process and curriculum style, clinical supervisors probably should not be too concerned about possible differences and should focus on what the particular curriculum requires and what their practice can offer. This could vary from quite specific demonstration and observation of clinical skills to allowing students to learn from experience with regular checking of progress. In most cases the approach of allowing the student to learn from guided experience and from seeking answers to questions remains appropriate.

Summary

This chapter has provided an overview of current curriculum development issues in order to explain where a practice attachment fits into a broader curriculum framework. Some curriculum content issues have been summarised, but clinical supervisors should read further on each of these issues should they wish to develop curriculum development expertise. Specific content issues are discussed where relevant to teaching and learning methods. The next chapter discusses the importance of assessment to clinical teaching.

Further reading

Allen I, Brown P and Hughes P (eds) (1997) *Choosing Tomorrow's Doctors*. London: Policy Studies Institute.

A series of papers that present contemporary views on what patients, governments and the profession itself expect from medical practitioners. Although written for a UK audience, the messages are reasonably global.

Elstein AS, Schulman LS and Sprafka SA (1978) *Medical Problem Solving: an analysis of clinical reasoning*. Cambridge, MA: Harvard University Press.

Almost the original seminal text explaining how doctors solve problems. Now an old book, but still worth reading.

General Medical Council (1997) *The New Doctor*. London: General Medical Council.

A contemporary description of how postgraduate education should be provided to medical graduates in the UK, but of relevance elsewhere. The booklet provides 39 principles of general medical training, along with the proposed duties of the organisers and teachers of postgraduate medical education and the responsibilities of postgraduate learners. This material has influenced the development of programmes that assess the performance of doctors who have been reported to the General Medical Council.

Schmidt HG, Norman GR and Boshuizen HPA (1990) A cognitive theory on medical expertise: theory and implications. *Academic Medicine*. **65**: 611–21.

A more recent explanation of clinical expertise and elaborated knowledge.

Stewart M, Brown JB, Weston WW, McWhinney IR, McWilliam CL and Freeman TR (1995) *Patient-Centered Medicine: transforming the clinical method*. Thousand Oaks, CA: Sage Publications, Inc.

Describes a more patient-centred approach to healthcare that requires GPs to involve patients in a partnership to reach agreement on the nature of health problems and of their management. This should improve compliance with management and also improve healthcare outcomes.

Chapter 3

Assessment of learning in general practice

> Examinations are formidable even to the best prepared, for the greatest fool may ask more than the wisest man can answer.
>
> Charles Caleb Colton, 1820

Clinical supervisors often feel uncomfortable when they are asked to assess the learners in their care. The nature of clinical supervision is that a bond develops between supervisor and learner. The longer the association, the more difficult it is for the supervisor to criticise their 'friend', the learner. Many supervisors prefer their learners to learn in a self-directed way, free of the constraints of what might be in an end-point examination. In a sense the curriculum is what comes through the door, and learners will gain from experience that is guided by an experienced clinician.

However, assessment is an integral part of teaching and learning. Indeed, it is probably the most important part. Supervisors are assessing their learners more or less continuously, even if these assessments are not formalised. This chapter provides a brief overview of current issues in educational assessment as a guide to general practitioners who teach or assess learners. It is written on the premise that the most important purpose of assessment is to assist learners to become competent professionals and it presents educational concepts and theory to support this. Information relevant to both practice-based and formal external assessments is presented, as clinical supervisors often act as examiners in formal examinations. Additional material is provided for those involved in formal examinations of clinical competence.

What is assessment?

Assessment could be defined as the measurement of achievement of progress towards meeting defined educational objectives. There are several different kinds of assessment, each with a different purpose. These are formative assessment, summative assessment and programme evaluation. A fourth variant is in-training assessment, which could be viewed as a hybrid of formative and summative assessment.

Formative assessment

Formative assessment is that which provides feedback to learners in order to guide progress. Many educational purists believe that this is the only worthwhile form of assessment, as it is unashamedly focused on the needs of individual learners who are negotiating their way through a curriculum. Individuals learn in different ways and at different rates, and formative assessment offers opportunities for self-paced assessment of progress towards goals. Learners can be open about their strengths and weaknesses and seek advice from educators. Results assist learners and educators to determine when 'mastery' of particular course objectives has been achieved and when remediation is required. Formative assessment is an essential part of any good educational programme. When performed correctly, few learners should be troubled by assessments at the end of courses.

Summative assessment

Summative assessment is that which indicates that a particular level of competence has been achieved at the end of either part, or all, of the educational programme. While it can provide useful feedback to learners (or candidates), this information might be too late to help candidates to progress beyond that particular point, unless they are required to retake the assessment. This decision-making role of summative assessment is responsible for the bad press accorded to examinations: nobody wants to fail. However, well-designed summative assessment, which is matched to course objectives and uses appropriate assessment methods, should fail only those with significant deficiencies.

Programme evaluation

Programme evaluation is assessment that indicates how well the course is meeting educational objectives. This is an infrequently discussed aspect of assessment, yet it is important. It is interesting that course organisers often blame unexpectedly poor assessment results on the learners ('a bad group'), when it is more likely that the course was not delivered appropriately or that the assessment was inappropriate.

In-training assessment

This is a form of continuous or progressive assessment that bridges gaps between formative and summative assessment approaches. Weaknesses of end-point summative assessment are that it assesses only a sample of the necessary knowledge, skills and attitudes and does this on only a single occasion, usually at the end of training. Not all of these attributes can be assessed in a formal examination, so it makes sense to assess some of these summatively during training. However, care must be taken to avoid interference with formative assessment, which is more important. Learners should be aware of the purpose of any assessments conducted during training, summative measures should be based on actual performance in the practice setting, feedback should still be given, and a flexible approach should be taken to timing and sequencing of summative assessments. In-training assessment is discussed in more detail elsewhere (Hays and Wellard, 1998).

Characteristics of good assessment practices

Assessment occurs in all health professional courses and comes in many forms. While there may be no such thing as 'perfect' assessment, good assessment should reflect the six characteristics listed in Box 3.1. All forms of assessment display these characteristics to a greater or lesser extent, and all are important. Sadly, much debate on assessment practices focuses on the first two, when a balanced approach to assessment should include consideration of all six.

> **Box 3.1 Characteristics of good assessment**
> * Validity
> * Reliability
> * Educational impact
> * Acceptability
> * Feasibility
> * Efficiency

The first characteristic is *validity*, or the capacity to assess that which is intended to be assessed. There are several kinds of validity, as listed in the glossary of terms (face validity, content validity, etc.), but all relate to measuring the correct attributes. Ideally, they relate to learning objectives of the particular course, which in turn reflect community and professional expectations. In the context of general practice, this means assessing those aspects of healthcare that do not normally take place in teaching hospitals. Issues such as the following should feature in assessment if they are part of the curriculum: the ability to work as part of a community-based team; the ability to understand the needs of patients with respect to their social, family and occupational issues; and a broader understanding of ethical and community values.

The second characteristic is *reliability*, or the capacity to produce the same result if the assessment is repeated. An important consideration is the potential conflict between validity and reliability. In theory, validity and reliability should both be high, but in practice many assessment methods regarded as having high validity demonstrate poor reliability. This is not, as some argue, because validity and reliability are opposing ends of the assessment spectrum, but rather because medical education research has not yet developed reliable methods of assessing some of those attributes now regarded as essential in primary care. However, while it is true to say that there is a tension between validity and reliability across the assessment spectrum, both are important.

The third characteristic is the *impact on the learning process* of students or candidates. Most will have heard the truism that 'assessment drives learning'. This is usually cited as a criticism of assessment. However, good assessment practices use this characteristic in a positive way by ensuring that they assess the right attributes (validity) using methods which reinforce learning processes. Remember that the assessed curriculum should be the same as the formal curriculum and the delivered curriculum (*see* Chapter 2).

The fourth is the *acceptability* of the assessment. This includes a range of community and professional ethical considerations that might have different emphases in certain contexts. For example, sending covert standardised patients is a powerful method of performance assessment that is acceptable in some countries, but not in others.

The fifth is *feasibility*, or the capacity for the assessment practices to consume resources, such as time, money and personnel. Many assessment practices are criticised because they are highly resource-intensive, but in reality most assessment methods occupy a great deal of time, space and other resources. In general, resource issues should not impede development of improved assessment practices, as it is likely that use of resources will simply change, rather than increase. However, some increase in resource utilisation is worthwhile if assessment improves substantially.

The sixth is *efficiency*, a psychometric property that indicates the capacity to produce an acceptable result with optimal use of examiners, test cases and particular test formats. The evaluation of assessment methods requires particular mathematical approaches that are not dealt with in any detail by this manual. A more detailed discussion of these attributes of assessment is suggested in the 'Further Reading' list below.

What is the standard?

Individuals are assessed against some kind of standard, which is used to determine a pass/fail decision and, often, grades of passes. An important question is: what is the most appropriate standard? Experienced assessors may have developed an intuitive understanding of what is an acceptable standard, but new assessors may need to think carefully through the issues in order to reach this point faster than experience alone allows.

Norm and criterion referencing

The first issue is the method of determining the appropriate standard. There are two broad approaches: norm referencing and criterion referencing. Norm referencing is comparison against the peer group. An example of this is a high-jump competition, where the winner is the one who jumps highest on the day, no matter what that height is. In terms of an examination paper, norm referencing sets the pass mark at (say) the bottom 10% (remember the bell-curve?). A 'distinction' could be awarded to candidates whose scores were in the top (say) 10% of scores. This means that decisions about grades and failing are made relative to the scores of all candidates at the particular examination, and that the proportion of failing candidates remains stable in all examinations. Another term for norm-referenced standards is relative standards.

The alternative approach is to determine standards for passing and grades that reflect what students should know. With this criterion-referencing approach, the pass rates may vary between examinations, reflecting the reality that all examination cohorts are unlikely to contain equal proportions of very bright or poor students. To return to the example of the high-jump competition, judges could determine that the gold medal would be awarded only if a height of 2.5 metres is achieved. Should no competitor achieve this, then no gold medal would be awarded. Alternatively, should two manage to clear this height, then two gold medals would be awarded. In terms of sporting competitions, this approach seems odd! Another term for criterion-referenced standards is absolute standards.

In terms of medical competence, it is important to ensure that all practitioners have achieved a particular level of competence. Hence, criterion referencing is the preferred approach in health educational assessment. However, criterion referencing is hard work, as it requires test developers to carefully consider how candidates should respond to the test items, either together or individually. It is important to do this correctly. There are a variety of approaches, none necessarily better than the others, and all possibly achieving slightly different results. Most use a combination of consensus by test item writers on the degree of difficulty, followed by quantitative analysis of the correct results for each item. For an excellent summary of the methods available, see Cusimano (1996).

Most so-called absolute standards include an element of relativity to the performance of others; indeed, most standard-setting methods are pragmatic, in that they include consideration of both relative and absolute approaches. However, be wary of standards that merely pretend to be criterion-referenced. For example, the pass mark could be set at (say) 60%, reflecting that 'our graduates must have demonstrated superior knowledge'. While this is presumably better than 50%, it is not particularly meaningful in the absence of information about how candidates should perform on each test item. Another 'pseudo' method is to set the pass mark at two standard deviations below the mean score. While this method is rational, in that it selects out only the bottom 2.5% of candidates, it still relates scores on individuals to those of the whole cohort.

A discussion of norm-referenced and criterion-referenced standards is probably more relevant to formal assessments of competence, such as an examination at the end of training, than to practice-based teaching. However, as evidence-based medicine assumes greater prominence in general practice, judgements about the progress of individual learners will increasingly reflect a rational, evidence-based understanding of how GPs should perform.

Levels of assessment

The second issue relevant to standards is the level of assessment. This is a multifaceted issue. First, consider whether the group to be tested is in the early part of the course or at the end. Clearly, those at the end of a course should achieve higher scores, when tested with the same test items. Hence, acceptable scores for test items used at multiple levels of assessment may be different. Assessment at particular levels of student progress may also require test items designed specifically for each level.

Second, consider whether the assessment intends to determine the competence or the performance of candidates. Competence reflects the level of what individuals can do under certain defined conditions. As a rule, competence is the most desirable level of assessment for candidates at the end of the course. Performance reflects what individuals do in their regular work, and has a closer relationship with healthcare outcomes. In reality it subsumes competence, as illustrated in Figure 3.1. It is difficult to imagine that an individual health practitioner could perform well without achieving competence, but the reverse is not necessarily true, as it is quite possible for an individual who has demonstrated competence at an examination to subsequently perform poorly. This should not be surprising, as the two are quite different. Performance assessment is the most desirable for professionals practising in the community, as we are interested in what actually happens. The significance of this distinction is that different assessment methods may be required for each level, as is illustrated in Figure 3.2, an adaptation of 'Miller's pyramid' (Miller, 1990).

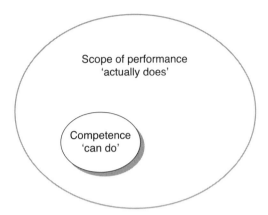

Figure 3.1 Relationship of competence to performance.

Third, consider how the assessment fits into professional hierarchies. Health professionals face several different levels of assessment, depending on their professional status. At the first level, as students, they are likely to be assessed on component knowledge and skills that, when combined, produce professional competence. At the end of their course they take competency examinations, which assess fitness to enter professional preparation courses. This level is often called 'licensure', particularly if there is a national competency assessment. Following professional preparation courses, they take more integrated clinical examinations, which measure fitness to enter unsupervised professional practice. This level is often called 'certification'. Following a period of supervised professional practice, they undertake assessments that demonstrate continuing fitness to practise. This 'recertification' assessment should be performance-based.

Finally, individuals with suspect poor performance may be required to undertake assessments, also performance based, which are used to diagnose deficiencies in order to plan remediation programmes. This perspective on professional assessment indicates how high the stakes can be in assessment of health professionals, particularly at the upper end. It is important to develop the best possible assessment programme, so that decisions are as correct as possible.

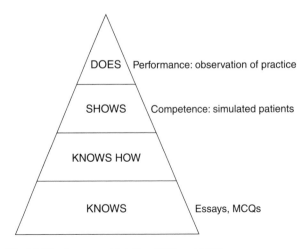

Figure 3.2 Modified Miller's pyramid (after Miller, 1990).

The relationship between curriculum and assessment

One of the main messages of this book is that assessment is an integral part of curriculum development. As discussed in Chapter 2, a curriculum must be the result of careful development, and should have explicit learning objectives that are linked to the content and processes of the curriculum. A curriculum should be expressed in the form of a blueprint, which acts as both a guide to learners and a rational guide to selection of what will be assessed.

Test blueprinting

To ensure that assessment reflects the curriculum, individual test items should reflect the components of competence in the curriculum blueprint, now called an assessment blueprint. Development of a blueprint is discussed further in Chapter 2. In theory, test items could come from any or all of the entries in Table 2.1. However, it is rarely feasible to assess everything in a curriculum, so test developers must sample components of competence for testing.

Sampling

There are usually time and resources for only a small proportion of the components of competence to be assessed, so determining which to assess is an important issue. Ideally, sampling of test items from a bank of items is done randomly, as this removes one form of bias from the assessment. So long as the test item bank has a sufficient number of good items, then random selection should produce a fair assessment of the 'universe'. Random selection can be done within domains, in order to ensure that the assessment reflects a particular weighting of domains. For example, should ethical issues be regarded as very important, test items with an ethical orientation could be over-sampled. However, beware of overdoing this. It is important to sample as widely as possible from all the 'components of competence', otherwise pass/fail decisions may be based on insufficient spread of the 'universe'.

A related issue is how to score items that assess 'critical' aspects of professional care. The temptation is to feel that 'if the candidate gets this question wrong, they should not be let loose on the public'! This concept is called the 'killer' question, a 'fatal flaw' or 'black-balling', and must be resisted. Instead, it has to be accepted that no professional gets every decision correct. There is an inbuilt error rate which cannot be corrected by examinations.

There are three ways to deal with this issue. The first is to assess 'essential' competencies prior to the formal examination. This makes those competencies 'hurdles' to achieve prior to assessment. For example, it could be argued that cardiopulmonary resuscitation skills are essential for all health professionals, so all should be certified as competent in these as part of training (and frequently thereafter, throughout a career!). The second is to ensure that the actual pass mark is criterion-referenced, through correct standard-setting procedures, as this takes into consideration what candidates should be able to achieve. The third is to ensure that all health professionals are skilled at self-directed learning, so that sound performance can be maintained throughout a career. Naturally, this is easier said than done.

Integrated assessment

A further interesting issue is whether to assess individual curriculum components (subjects or domains) or the integration of those individual components. As a rule, the higher the level of the assessment (as in Figure 3.2), the more appropriate it is to assess in an integrated manner. Naturally, proponents of problem-based learning would disagree with this, preferring to teach and assess in an integrated manner from day one.

Particularly with professional practice, the most desirable method is to assess how individuals perform in the workplace. As professional practice requires integration of a range of domains of knowledge, skills and attitudes, it makes little sense to assess these individually. Professional practice in primary care is about dealing with real people and real problems, so the more the assessment focuses on these issues, the better. Writing integrated test items is not difficult, but requires teachers of particular parts of the course to accept that it is possible to assess their particular parts indirectly, as a building block of professional practice.

Who should assess?

The traditional model of medical education has learners being taught and assessed by medical practitioners. While only another medical practitioner in the same discipline can judge many of the attributes of competent practice, the profession is not the only group with views on what determines quality of care. In particular, contemporary general practice requires proficient teamwork and consideration of the views of Government and consumers (Consumer Health Forum, 1996). Consumers are often in a better position to assess communication skills and humanitarian aspects of care, and should have a role in the assessment of general practitioners (Greco *et al.*, 1998).

Common forms of practice-based assessment

Medical education employs many different assessment methods, including multiple-choice questions (MCQs), written tests (short and long answer, and a more recent development called Key Feature Problems [KFPs]), and clinical assessment methods. In this book the focus in on the latter, as GP supervisors will not often get involved in writing and scoring written tests. Any who are interested in doing so should contact the educational institution, which will embrace them wholeheartedly!

Clinical assessment in general practices has the advantage of being workplace based and performance oriented (higher up Miller's pyramid). Here it is possible to assess what the learners actually do in clinical practice, and for GP registrars this is very close indeed to future practice. Commonly used assessment methods include: observing consultations in real time; observing videotaped consultations; patient feedback; and reviewing patient records, referrals, prescribing and referral patterns. In all cases the supervisor is asked to make a judgement about learner performance. This will more often be for formative assessment, but can (perhaps more likely in the future) be summative. Whatever the purpose, the judgement should be based on detailed knowledge of what the learner should be able to achieve at their level (i.e. the standard), and recorded appropriately with a combination of quantitative (i.e. a score) and qualitative (written feedback) data.

Individual assessment methods are discussed in subsequent chapters, where they are presented primarily as learning methods. A brief description of the scoring issues is provided here.

Use of assessment instruments

Some assessments need to be formal, as they count towards career progression. Even when they do not, it is a good idea to document strengths and weaknesses in order to provide more comprehensive feedback. There are two ways of scoring performance: an attribute is either present or absent (dichotomous scoring); or there are degrees of performance quality from 0 or 1 (not at all) to a number (say, 5). These kinds of assessment instruments have particular applications.

Checklists

A simple form of assessment is to determine a list of what should happen and record whether or not each one did. This is commonly used in observing consultations. For example, an observer might have a checklist like the example in Figure 3.3 to guide observation and provision of feedback. This could be a generic checklist, used in all situations but filled in only where relevant, or it could be designed specifically for each assessment item (the preferred approach). There might be some information to identify the consultation and then lists of activities or behaviours that might be desirable. Precise headings would have to be specific to the presenting complaint. If the assessment were formal, then a score could be derived by adding up the 'ticks' as a score out of the total number of possible ticks. Clearly, this would need careful consideration and standard setting by the question-writing team (see earlier in this chapter).

Age: *4y 8m*	**Gender:** *m*		**Duration:** *13'30"*
Presenting complaint: *fever 48 hours, pulling ears*			
Communication skills:			
Empathic	Spoke to child		Explained well
History:			
Vomiting	Diarrhoea	Appetite	Fluids
Urine output	Siblings	Vaccinations	
Examination:			
Ears Throat	Chest	Abdo	Hydration
Neck stiffness	Drowsiness		Rashes
Investigations:			
WTU			
Differential:			
URTI	Otitis media	Pharyngitis	Meningitis
Correct diagnosis:			
Otitis media			
Management:			
Fluids	Paracetamol		Antibiotics???

Figure 3.3 Possible checklist for observing consultations.

Rating scales

Rating scales require a judgement to be made about the degree to which an attribute was exhibited. There is usually a sliding scale with points that indicate degrees of quality of performance. There are two kinds of scale. The first uses numbers to indicate the intervals, from 1 (absent) to a number indicating perfect, usually from 5 to 10. This is called a Likert scale. Sometimes the polarity of the scales is reversed, such that 1 means excellent and 5 means absent. This is sometimes done to detect scorers who tend to rate globally (see below), but can be confusing. Numerical scales are easy to use, but they are often misused in formal scoring. They cannot really be added to produce a total numerical score unless there are at least 10 interval points, as measurement theory does not regard the intervals to be equal.

The second kind uses verbal descriptors to define intervals; terms such as 'extremely poor', 'poor', 'acceptable', 'very good' and 'excellent' are commonly used. These are called semantic differential scales. They are also easy to use, but are usually poorly developed. The descriptors should describe, as well as is feasible, the actual behaviour which merits that rating. The use of 'very poor' to 'excellent' is meaningless unless more information, called 'behavioural anchors', is provided for each heading. Behavioural anchors are also sometimes used with Likert scales. Examples of both numerical and semantic differential scales are provided in Figure 3.4.

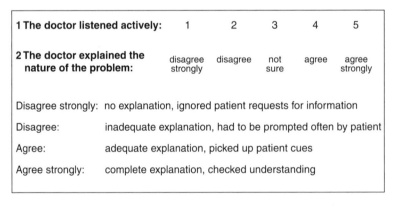

Figure 3.4 Examples of numerical and semantic differential rating scales.

Common pitfalls to avoid in the use of rating scales include:

- Central tendency marking (Figure 3.5a). This is where assessors tend to score consistently at about the middle score, rather than using the full range of scores. Performance is often good in places and poor in others, so score it that way.
- Halo effect (Figure 3.5b). This is where an assessor allows judgement of one aspect of performance to affect judgement of other aspects. If the learner is a 'nice' person, it might be difficult to assess them poorly; the reverse is also true for learners who are thought to be not nice people. Scores should use different intervals for different aspects of performance.
- Black-balling (Figure 3.5c). This is where an assessor decides that poor performance in one aspect equals an automatic overall fail, regardless of how well other aspects are performed.

- Being a 'dove' (Figure 3.5d). This kind of assessor scores everybody highly.
- Being a 'hawk' (Figure 3.5e). This kind of assessor scores everybody poorly.
- Failure to observe. Assessment requires concentration, which can lapse because of fatigue. Assessors should not have to observe more than about seven or eight similar interactions without a break.

Instead, assessors should try to rate each item on a rating scale independently, based on a realistic estimation of how learners should perform for that aspect. Correct standard setting and calibration of assessors (through training and experience) produces better scoring.

a Central tendency scoring

Correct questions were asked	1	2	3	4	5
Differential diagnoses were appropriate	1	2	3	4	5
Investigations were appropriate	1	2	3	4	5
Correct management options explored	1	2	3	4	5
Patient explanation was adequate	1	2	3	4	5
Overall performance was adequate	1	2	3	4	5

b Halo marking

Correct questions were asked	1	2	3	4	5
Differential diagnoses were appropriate	1	2	3	4	5
Investigations were appropriate	1	2	3	4	5
Correct management options explored	1	2	3	4	5
Patient explanation was adequate	1	2	3	4	5
Overall performance was adequate	1	2	3	4	5

c Black-balling

Correct questions were asked	1	2	3	4	5	
Differential diagnoses were appropriate	1	2	3	4	5	
Investigations were appropriate	1	2	3	4	5	
Correct management options explored	1	2	3	4	5	*FAIL!!*
Patient explanation was adequate	1	2	3	4	5	
Overall performance was adequate	1	2	3	4	5	

d 'Dovish' marking

Correct questions were asked	1	2	3	4	5
Differential diagnoses were appropriate	1	2	3	4	5
Investigations were appropriate	1	2	3	4	5
Correct management options explored	1	2	3	4	5
Patient explanation was adequate	1	2	3	4	5
Overall performance was adequate	1	2	3	4	5

e 'Hawkish' marking

Correct questions were asked	1	2	3	4	5
Differential diagnoses were appropriate	1	2	3	4	5
Investigations were appropriate	1	2	3	4	5
Correct management options explored	1	2	3	4	5
Patient explanation was adequate	1	2	3	4	5
Overall performance was adequate	1	2	3	4	5

Figure 3.5 Examples of common pitfalls in using rating scales.
(5 = disagree strongly; 4 = disagree; 3 = unsure; 2 = agree; 1 = agree strongly)

Summary

This chapter has presented an overview of current issues in assessment in medical education. Understanding of these issues is important because assessment is such an integral part of education. The most important reason to assess learners is to guide learning. Each assessment should reflect a judgement about a score on each item, rather than being contaminated by judgements about other items. It is uncommon for learners to score equally highly in all assessment items, and it is important to provide accurate information about those differences. When making assessments, supervisors should provide as much information about the performance of learners as possible, as this is the basis of the feedback provided. The next six chapters build on the concepts and theory of the last two chapters to provide much more practical discussions of how to provide practice-based teaching that is both interesting and educationally sound.

Further reading

Best JW and Kahn JV (1989) *Research in Education* (5e). Englewood Cliffs, NJ: Prentice-Hall.
An overview of approaches to educational research and evaluation. Full of practical examples from classroom settings. Presents clear descriptions of how to create rating scales.

Cusimano MD (1996) Standard setting in medical education. *Academic Medicine.* **71** (Suppl.): S112–20.
A comprehensive overview of current approaches to setting standards in assessment that explains complex methods in a practical, more reader-friendly way.

Greco M, Francis W, Buckley J, Brownlea A and McGovern J (1998) Real patient evaluation of communication skills teaching for GP registrars. *Family Practice.* **15** (1): 51–7.
An example of how patients' views can be assessed and used as formative assessment for learners. The method has been validated and trialled in several contexts.

Hays RB and Wellard R (1998) In-training assessment in postgraduate training for general practice. *Medical Education.* **32**: 307–12.
This paper presents a conceptual framework for maintaining the roles of formative and summative assessment during training. Both are necessary, but for different purposes. The most important for learning is formative, but summative assessment demonstrates to the community that competence has been achieved. Some of the latter can be conducted during training.

Miller GE (1990) The assessment of clinical skills/competence/performance. *Academic Medicine.* **65** (Suppl.): S563–7.
This paper presents a conceptual framework that explains the need to assess what doctors do as close as possible to actual practice conditions. This principle has driven research and development in assessment for the last ten years.

Van der Vleuten CPM (1996) The assessment of professional competence: developments, research and practical implications. *Advances in Health Sciences Education.* **1**: 41–67.
An authoritative overview of the principles of assessment applied to health professions.

Chapter 4

Teaching and learning in action

> We do not receive wisdom. We must discover it for ourselves after experience which no one else can have for us and from which no one can spare us.
>
> Marcel Proust, 1918

The previous two chapters have dealt with some of the conceptual and theoretical aspects of clinical practice-based supervision. Now it is time to place this theory into a practical framework for application. Learning in practice attachments is more or less inevitable. The challenge for clinical supervisors is to guide learners through a tangle of competing needs and time pressures towards achieving mastery of agreed learning objectives that reflect the curriculum, the opportunities afforded by the practice and the personal aims of the learner.

Models of teaching and learning

One way of thinking about teaching and learning is to consider the degree of responsibility that lies with both the teacher and the learner. One form of teaching is the direct passage of information from expert to novice – traditional didactic teaching. Some cruelly call this the 'jug to mug' approach. It has its place in certain circumstances, although it can be overdone. Just think about most medical school curricula, which include so many lectures that little opportunity is left for independent learning. These curricula also assume that learners should follow similar pathways (content, process and sequencing) to achieve the desired level of learning, when there is little evidence to support this. A further disadvantage is that information acquired this way is easily forgotten, as it is often not provided in a clinically meaningful way. However, early in the progress of learning, there is a place for 'priming' learners to start them on a more self-directed approach. At key points in learning acquisition, learners might benefit from a condensed overview of current issues that might reinforce or redirect learning. An example of this is the liking that general practitioners have for short lectures from acknowledged experts on clinical topics. If delivered well, they can offer a current clinical perspective that is not available elsewhere.

A second model is problem-based learning. This approach integrates basic and clinical science curriculum strands and themes into clinical problems, which are simulated clinical scenarios constructed carefully to encourage learners to discover knowledge and skills that are relevant to the clinical scenario. Learners are more independent and may learn more from each other than from their teachers. There is evidence that knowledge is remembered better this way, as it is recalled when learners are confronted later by similar clinical scenarios. A further potential advantage is that it might produce more self-directed learners, but there is little evidence to support this. An appropriate learning environment that provides access to textbooks, journals, electronic databases and 'experts' must support problem-based learning. Information management systems can assist this. A range of individual teaching methods may be employed, including some didactic teaching at key points. This model is arguably more resource-intensive and is difficult to apply to large cohorts of learners, and is not usually applied to more advanced clinical learning.

A third model is that used in medical school clinical rotations and vocational training. This is apprenticeship-based clinical teaching that combines a less explicitly defined curriculum, learning by doing and a substantial amount of formative assessment. Learners are allowed a degree of choice about what to learn, particularly at more advanced levels. A wide range of learning methods is used, according to learning style and learning objectives. Teachers are really supervisors, guiding and nurturing learning.

A fourth model is true independent, self-directed learning. This is the traditional model of continuing medical education, where learners choose what, how and when to learn, and take complete responsibility for their maintenance of competence.

These models of teaching could be placed along a spectrum of responsibility for learning, as in Figure 4.1. This places the third model, clinical supervision, towards the right, where responsibility is still shared but is predominantly with the learner. This model is more fully explored later in this chapter.

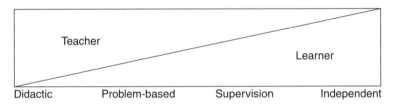

Figure 4.1 Locus of responsibility for learning for four models of teaching.

How do learners learn?

Reflect for a moment on your preferred learning methods. Do you remember more after reading, being told what to do by a more senior colleague, listening to audiotapes, watching videotapes or by just 'doing'? If you think that your preferred learning methods are the same as those of other health professionals, you might be in for a surprise. While there is some evidence that members of health professional groups tend to have similar learning styles, individual learning styles may vary widely. Most health professionals prefer to learn from interaction and discussion with colleagues and from practising new skills in clinical practice. Some learn well from reading journals and books, whereas for others this has a similar effect to sleeping pills. Some like to understand why certain things happen – an analytical approach – whereas others are just happy to know that things happen.

It might be useful to formally explore learning styles, both your own and those of your learners. Some interesting self-completion questionnaires are available to assist this. The first is a learning styles questionnaire, which was developed by Honey and Mumford (1986), and applied to healthcare professionals by Lewis and Bolden (1989). The second is a self-directed learning questionnaire, as used by Bligh (1993). They are fun to do and can provoke interesting discussions with colleagues and students. Although the results are not necessarily foolproof, these are useful 'ice-breaker' exercises that can lead to valuable discussions and raising of self-awareness.

Learning knowledge, skills and attitudes

Educators often divide components of learning into knowledge, skills and attitude domains, as this helps us to understand that learning must incorporate *what* to do, *how* to do it, and *when, where* and *why* to do it. These domains are different not only conceptually, but also in their optimal learning modes. Whereas knowledge can be acquired through reading and listening to lectures, skills should be observed and practised, and attitudes are best adopted through role-modelling.

Practice-based teaching does not include lectures. Instead, learners come to a practice attachment with some knowledge, skills and attitudes learned in other settings. What they now need are opportunities to see knowledge applied in context, to observe and practise clinical skills, and to adopt appropriate professional behaviour through observation of doctors with high ethical and attitudinal standards.

Contextual learning

All learning is best achieved in the right context or setting. A simple example is that general practice is better learned in general practice that in hospitals. However, there are many different kinds of general practice, and some desirable learning objectives are learned better in particular kinds of general practice settings. For example, the achievement of an understanding of different cultures, values and belief systems is more likely if learners are immersed in those cultures. There are two broad categories of different 'cultures' that are topical in Australian medical education – indigenous health and rural/remote health. Learners should be placed in practice attachments where people of the desired culture are encountered frequently and the health professionals observed role-model desirable professional and ethical approaches to their management. It sounds almost too obvious that rural practice should be learned in rural practice attachments and that indigenous healthcare should be learned in indigenous healthcare practices. However, this is worth stating, because not all educational organisations demonstrate understanding of this basic principle.

Adult learning

Conceptually, adult learning means allowing learners greater choice of, and control over, what and how they will learn. Adult learners are regarded as experienced in life, with prior experiences that can facilitate learning. They should be able to commence an educational programme that is relevant to past experiences, current level of knowledge and future directions. Learning is essentially experiential.

The principles of adult learning can be briefly stated as being:

- learners value the learning activities
- learners take responsibility for their learning
- learners like to receive feedback on their performance
- learners should be challenged to solve problems that are relevant to future roles
- learners value time for reflection and independent learning
- learners require opportunities to practise acquired knowledge and experience, that is, they must build on experience
- learners are free to make mistakes and to learn from them.

Attributes of a 'good' teacher

In adult learning, different learning styles are better suited to different teaching styles, so what one person would define as a good teacher, another might classify as a poor teacher. Similarly, some learning activities will appear to the teacher to be more effective than others. However, in general, learners look for teachers who are friendly, cheerful, sympathetic, enthusiastic and humorous. Effective teachers are fair and democratic, responsive and understanding, original and entertaining, and alert and confident (*see* Table 4.1).

Table 4.1 Attributes of effective and ineffective teachers

Effective	*Ineffective*
Fair and democratic	Autocratic and aloof
Responsive and understanding	Restricted and dull
Original and entertaining	Harsh and evasive
Alert and confident	Erratic and excitable

This requires further elaboration for practice-based clinical supervision. Teachers in a 'real-life' general practice are also senior colleagues who often must trust the judgement of their learner, who might collect information and make clinical decisions on behalf of the practice. The extent to which the junior colleague is relied upon depends on the level of the learner, and is higher with GP registrars than with medical students. Practice-based supervisors are managers of an apprenticeship, which is a wider role than simply teaching the 'right way to do it'. Current literature on the supervision and teaching of professionals organises supervision duties into six roles: manager; counsellor; instructor; observer; the giver of feedback; and evaluator. These roles are not always clear-cut, and many times will merge together during the teaching of professionals. It is no wonder that clinical supervisors could benefit from training!

A process of collaborative supervision

The effectiveness of a supervisor will depend on how many of the above-mentioned traits can be demonstrated to the learner. Collaborative supervision is a process that has been developed to assist this complex task. The features of this process include:

- a basic premise that professional practice can only be improved by direct feedback on issues that are of concern to the learner
- understanding that the relationship between learner and supervisor is critical. Ideally, supervisors are regarded as trusted colleagues, rather than as teachers
- learner-centredness, focusing on the learner's strengths and weaknesses
- self-reflection on practice to increase self-awareness of performance
- implementing and monitoring change in practice behaviour
- role-modelling of supervisors demonstrating the knowledge, skills and attitudes that learners are expected to achieve.

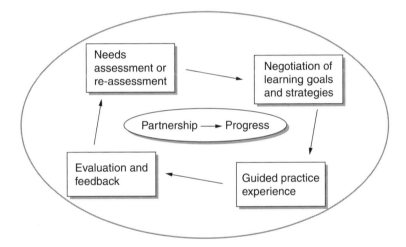

Figure 4.2 A collaborative supervision model for teaching and learning.

The process of collaborative supervision could be seen as a three-stage process of need-based negotiation, implementation and evaluation, as shown in Figure 4.2. All stages involve learners and supervisors as partners. This process underpins the entire clinical attachment and each learning activity during the attachment. This cycle should be repeated many times during an attachment, as goals are achieved and new goals are developed. Hence, clinical supervision is a highly planned, though flexible, approach that meets the identified needs of the learner.

Negotiation of learning needs

This phase is critical to the success of the clinical attachment. Just as one would not increase a dose of digoxin without first knowing the serum digoxin level, supervisors should not either provide education that might be unnecessary or unwanted, or omit education because of an incorrect assumption that it was unnecessary. Learners and supervisors should meet either prior to, or at the commencement of, the attachment, to jointly plan the learning objectives and learning strategies for the attachment. An example of part of an early planning meeting is provided in Box 4.1. The learner should be encouraged to state their expectations, while remaining aware of the requirements of the curriculum, by a patient supervisor who uses open questions. The process is not much different to exploring a patient's agenda during a consultation.

Planning should consider curriculum objectives provided by the educational institution, the personal progress and needs of the learner, and the opportunities offered by the particular practice and supervisor, as documented in a practice teaching plan (see below). Some form of learning plan should be developed and preferably documented for future use. The plan should identify: specific learning objectives, appropriate learning strategies, and methods of knowing that those objectives have been achieved. The nature of the learning objectives will depend on the level of the learner, as discussed in Chapter 2.

As an example, an undergraduate student will probably have an overall goal of gaining a broad understanding of what the particular health professional does in his or her practice. At the other end of the spectrum, an advanced postgraduate learner is likely to need quite specific, higher-level knowledge, skills or attitudes to 'round off' training. Examples of learning plans for both a less advanced and a more advanced learner are provided in Box 4.2. Such learning plans are not set in concrete, but should be revised as often as necessary by further joint meetings that review learning progress during the attachment.

Box 4.1 Extract from an early planning meeting with a supervisor (S) and learner (L)

S. It's great to have you here John. As you know, we have taken a lot of medical students and we really enjoy the challenge of seeing you develop. I would be interested to know just why you chose our practice.

L. The medical school keeps a book with information about all of the practices that take students. I live not far from here and went through the list of practices in this area. I was impressed with the feedback that past students have given this practice. They all seem to have had an enjoyable time. I was also particularly interested in the acupuncture part of this practice. I have not seen it done before, but have heard a lot about it.

S. Well thanks for the feedback. I wish the medical school would give us more feedback about what we do. So, acupuncture. Well, of course you can see that while you are here, but there might be other things to cover in just two weeks. You are in your first really clinical year, so there might be some basic GP issues that are worth covering. The medical school has sent me a guide – have you read that?

L. Yes and most of that is fine. But I am almost at the end of the year, and so I think that I have covered some of it in my hospital terms.

S. So, what do you think are the main priorities?

L. I would like to see as wide a range of clinical problems as possible while I am here. I have heard from students in earlier terms that some see some really fascinating and unusual things, while others seem to see just colds and things like that. Of course, I have already mentioned acupuncture, and I would also like to do some procedures, like suturing, if possible.

S. Your friends have described general practice in all its diversity! It varies from being mundane to being really exciting. Every week I see patients that really excite my interest, so I will have to make sure that you can be part of that. Procedures are a little different, as this is a private practice in a city. Therefore we do only a limited range of procedures and have to have the consent of the patient for a student to perform them. However, I am happy to negotiate that with patients for you – which procedures in particular are you thinking of?

The negotiation of learning does not stop with this early planning meeting. It is possible that the objectives for the attachment will not be achievable in the designated time-frame. Learners often identify rather ambitious learning objectives or, particularly with less experienced learners, may not be able to focus on specific objectives until some time into the attachment. The desired clinical caseload may not eventuate, particularly for learning procedural skills. Hence it is sensible to regularly review the learning plan and ask the questions: 'Is this being achieved? If not, how can we change either the plan or what we do in the practice to make the plan achievable?' With longer attachments, it is desirable to hold brief, regular weekly meetings with the learner to review progress. In addition, a more formal meeting half way through the attachment and one towards the end of the term, so that deviations from the agreed plan can be monitored and addressed.

Box 4.2 Examples of typical learning plans for practice attachments for learners in both early and late vocational training

a. Earlier attachment
Gain a broad understanding of what general practice is like
Practise communication skills
Learn how community GPs work with the hospital system
Learn about prescribing in private practice
Gain experience with removing skin lesions

b. Later attachment
Gain further experience in certain (e.g. simple skin flap) procedures
Gain more confidence in community palliative care
Become involved in practice management
Prepare for the examination!

A practice teaching plan

All teaching practices should develop a practice teaching plan that guides practice-based teaching and learning. This is a kind of teaching–learning 'master plan' that must be adapted for individual learners and attachments. Such a plan could include:

- descriptions of the practice: location, layout, staff and service provision arrangements
- descriptions of the practice population, community links, local health needs and priorities, e.g. age, gender, disease profiles, local industry, etc.
- descriptions of teaching resources available in the practice: staff responsible for teaching, their clinical and educational interests, library and internet access, etc.
- strengths and opportunities offered by the practice to learners, e.g. sports medicine, women's health, palliative care, etc. This information should reflect practice and staff profiles
- how teaching and learning are organised in the practice. For example, what teaching methods are used, when and how often supervisors and learners meet, who is available to assist with particular needs, etc.
- what assessments are made and how they are made.

This information is useful for three reasons. First, the development of a practice teaching plan assists both supervisors and their practices to become teaching oriented. Teaching and learning are active processes that require thought and planning. Second, it helps learners to select practices on the basis of the quality of the clinical and educational experience. Particular attributes of practices, such as scope of clinical work encountered and interests of staff, can be matched to the prior needs and interests of learners. Third, this information is useful for evaluation of teaching in practices, as teaching plans help set parameters against which performance might be measured. This role in the evaluation of teaching and learning is discussed in Chapter 12. An example of a practice teaching plan is provided in Box 4.3.

Broad principles of clinical teaching

The following chapters provide details on a range of practice-based teaching methods. These include direct observation of practice by sitting in, audiotape or videotape review, one-to-one clinical topic tutorials, and review of written records and projects. All of these methods employ common principles of clinical teaching, as follows:

- Learning should occur in the context of real clinical encounters. Knowledge without application is relatively useless. This is the basis of 'case-based' teaching and learning. Learners will remember better when they are able to reflect on past examples. The more they see and learn, the more diagnoses will be based on elaborated knowledge (pattern matching) rather than hypothetico-deductive (*see* Chapter 2). Expertise is built through experience.
- Learning should be inquiry-based. Experience alone is not enough. Experience will generate questions for which learners seek answers. However, learners will remember better when they personally discover information and skills relevant to their practice. Supervisors should resist the temptation to provide quick answers to questions. It is often better to turn the question back to the learner, suggesting that they find out the answer and tell you at a future

appointment. This is the 'educational prescription' concept developed by Sackett (1997).

Box 4.3 A simple practice teaching plan for a GP registrar

Drs Wendy Smith & Susan Jones
12 Green St, Harley
Phone: (05)123 45678
Fax: (05)876 54321
Email: Susan.Jones@email.address

Welcome to your clinical attachment at our practice. We would like you to enjoy the experience and gain as much as possible from it.

The practice. This is a busy three-doctor practice in an outer suburb of a growing town. The surgery is open from 8.30 am to 6.30 pm Monday–Friday and from 8.30 am to 12 pm Saturday. There are three consulting rooms, a nurse's room, a treatment room and a spare room that acts as a small practice library/tea room. We care for about 3000 patients, including people of all ages and with a wide range of problems. We have an arrangement with the nearby textile mill to provide occupational health services. Most patients are seen by appointment, but the system accommodates urgent fit-ins on the day. We normally see about 300 patients per week. The practice is part of an after-hours collective of 30 local GPs.

The staff. Dr Wendy Smith has been in the practice for 15 years. Her special interests are counselling and aged care. Dr Susan Jones has been here for 8 years and tends towards child health and women's health. The third doctor is a GP registrar. The receptionist is Jeremy Taylor and the practice nurse is Jenny Brown.

Teaching and learning. This has been a teaching practice for 4 years. Dr Jones is the primary supervisor, although all staff participate in teaching. The practice offers opportunities to learn from a wide range of patients and presentations, but offers particular opportunities in counselling, aged care, child health, women's health and occupational health. We also like all of our learners to spend time with both the receptionist and the practice nurse. The surgery will not be the only place of learning, as learners will attend visits to patients' homes, nursing homes, hospitals and the textile mill. Learners will also participate in after-hours care. We keep a small number of current journals and books in the spare room for use as required.

Learners spend the first session sitting in with Dr Jones. This is to help orient you to the practice and to plan the rest of the stay. You will be expected to meet with Dr Jones every Wednesday and Friday afternoon, between 1 pm to 3 pm, to discuss issues as they arise and to work through some of the topics provided by the course organiser. A list of these can be found on the tea room notice board. Please look at these and let us know what your priorities are. During your time here, you will have access to a video camera and player, and we would like you to record some consultations for discussion with Dr Jones. The tea room also has a PC with internet access; feel free to use it as required.

Teaching timetable for week 1:					
Monday	*Tuesday*	*Wednesday*	*Thursday*	*Friday*	*Saturday*
am. With Dr Jones	Consulting	Consulting	Consulting	Consulting	Consulting (every third)
pm. With Dr Smith	Consulting	1–3 Tutorial Consulting	Registrar meeting	1–3 Tutorial then free	

- Learning should be reflective. Asking questions of learners is a powerful way of providing feedback and directing learning. Learners should be encouraged to question themselves often, and seek answers to those questions. Where possible, answers should be evidence-based.
- Learning should be supported by a range of relevant and useful educational resources that are held within the practice. Some suggestions for a teaching practice 'library' are provided in the Appendix.
- Learning should involve longitudinal involvement in clinical care. One of the differences between general practice and hospital-based disciplines is that care is provided over a period of time. With longer attachments, the concept of continuity of care can be understood from personal experience. However, even with short attachments, learners can participate on a learning journey that touches on several aspects and involves several providers of care. A simple technique is to attach learners to patients who are referred to specialists or hospitals. By observing and participating in what happens as patients negotiate their way from initial presentation, through investigations, referral, treatment and back to the general practitioner, learning can be quite powerful.
- Learning occurs through role-modelling. This is remarkably powerful. Just as Balint spoke of the doctor as the 'drug' (Balint, 1986), meaning that doctors can have profound effects on their patients, so supervisors can have profound effects on their learners. Clinicians often talk about particular individuals who had a profound influence on their careers. Ideally, supervisors should demonstrate a reflective, inquiry-based learning style to their learners. This role-models good learning behaviour for the next generation of teachers.

Teaching methods and levels of learners

Just as curriculum content is dependent on the level of learning, some teaching and learning methods are more appropriate to different levels of learning. For example, while the above principles of learning (and tools such as educational prescriptions and patient tracking) can be applied at any level, the methods presented in the following chapters are more suited to particular levels of learning. The more 'invasive' methods, which involve learners taking active roles in patient management, are clearly more suited to postgraduate learners. However, no method is exclusively linked to any level, as even less advanced learners can benefit from being 'in control' for parts of consultations and procedures. It is just that they will do this less often than more advanced learners.

This is reflected in Table 4.2. The application of particular teaching and learning strategies will be discussed in the following chapters.

Table 4.2 Teaching and learning methods and levels of learning

	Less advanced	*More advanced*
Simple observation of Dr	+++	+
Simple observation of learner	+	++
Conjoint consultation	+	+++
Audiotape review	++	+
Videotape review	+	+++
Written record review	+	+++
Projects and audits	++	+++

Contextualised learning

One of the great debates in recent Australian medical education has focused on how to teach rural, rather than urban, general practice. While this debate has been loud and remains largely unresolved at a political level, the issues are really quite simple.

There is substantial evidence that GPs in rural and urban primary care encounter a largely similar case-load, at least as this is defined by presenting complaint. Further, potential diagnoses encountered are similar. However, the diagnostic work-up and the management may well be different, depending on the degree of professional isolation of the doctor's practice.

Rural doctors also do see some different clinical content, mainly in the areas of public health and more urgent (often after-hours) medicine. Further, although there are wide variations in scope and depth of practice, some rural doctors in more remote areas provide procedural skills normally provided by urban specialists. The islands off Scotland are the clearest UK example, but the mountains in a wintry Wales pose similar challenges to transporting the sick. In the UK, rural and urban GPs have elected to work together, both academically and politically, whereas in Australia there is a strong difference in opinion, resulting in a poor collaboration.

The relevance of this debate is that in medical education, context is important. The best way for learners to learn about rural practice is for them to be immersed in rural practice, encountering rural patients, participating in their care and observing rural medical role models. Similarly, learning about indigenous health is best in indigenous health centres, where Australian Aboriginal, Torres Strait Islander or Maori cultures and healthcare models are encountered. Within those contexts, the theory and practice of teaching and learning are similar.

When the supervisor–learner relationship goes wrong

Sometimes, when two individuals form a supervisor–learner relationship, which is often close, the relationship proves not to be constructive. The usual cause of this is a clash of personalities. This should not be seen as a fault of either the supervisor or the learner, although a record of several similar clashes might lead course organisers to conclude that either the supervisor or the learner has a deeper problem, which might need to be diagnosed and addressed. The more difficult problems are usually due to poor attitudes or mental health concerns, but there is evidence that many GP registrars find their training stressful, balancing personal and professional demands and coping with relocation for training positions (Larkins *et al.*, 2004).

When the relationship does not work out, the supervisor should recognise this and take action. Depending on the severity of the problem, this might be a frank discussion of the matter with the learner. This discussion should acknowledge that a problem exists and explore ways of retrieving educational value. Should the matter not be resolved within the practice, the supervisor should inform the course organiser, who should make an assessment of the situation. Should this assessment indicate that a resolution is unlikely, the learner should be moved to another supervisor, still on a 'no fault' premise. It is far better to start again than to try to patch up a poor relationship between learner and supervisor. Sometimes the situation can become quite destructive for both the progress of the learner and the enthusiasm of the supervisor.

Such situations can be difficult for all concerned. No matter how friendly a supervisor–learner relationship might be, it is still a relationship between a teacher and a learner, with an obvious imbalance of power within the educational organisation. Hence the main responsibility for taking action rests with the supervisor, although learners will also be encouraged to report problems to the course organiser.

Summary

This chapter has presented material that should help supervisors better understand the teaching and learning processes involved in clinical supervision. While the model risks being seen as highly idealised, it is practical to implement in even busy clinical practices. The next chapters present practical discussions of how to apply particular teaching and learning strategies in busy general practices.

Further reading

Hall M, Dwyer D and Lewis T (1999) *The GP Training Handbook.* Oxford: Blackwell Science.
  A blend of educational theory and general practice structure and organisation from the perspective of the UK National Health Service.
Knowles M (1990) *The Adult Learner: a neglected species* (4e). Houston, TX: Gulf Publishing Company.
  The original book about adult learning. Very theoretical, perhaps more for those wanting to delve more deeply.
Mohanna K, Wall D and Chambers R (2004) *Teaching Made Easy: a manual for health professionals.* Oxford: Radcliffe Publishing.
  Despite the misleading name (teaching is not so easy!), this provides a more detailed description of how to implement adult learning theory within a multi-professional healthcare context.
Newble D and Cannon R (2001) *A Handbook for Clinical Teachers* (4e). Dordrecht: Kluwer Academic Publishers.
  A practical guide to how to run educational events, mostly at undergraduate level.

Schon D (1991) *The Reflective Practitioner: how professionals think in action.* Aldershot: Ashgate Publishing Ltd. (1991 reprint.)

Describes engagingly how professional people learn by doing.

Verduin JR, Miller HG and Greer CE (1997) *Adults Teaching Adults: principles and strategies.* TX: Learning Concepts.

Another book bridging theory and practice, from a North American perspective.

Whitman N (1990) *Creative Medical Teaching.* Salt Lake City, Utah: Department of Family and Preventive Medicine, University of Utah School of Medicine.

Full of innovative and interesting teaching and learning strategies, including games and fun activities that are ideal as ice breakers and learning enhancers. Most are designed for group learning, but a little adaptation makes many strategies ideal for one-to-one supervision.

Whitman N and Schwenk TL (1997) *The Physician as Teacher* (2e). Salt Lake City, Utah: Whitman Associates.

Simple and readable book about teaching in clinical settings, although these are usually in-patient settings.

Chapter 5

Sitting in

> Man is essentially the imitative animal. His whole educability and in
> fact the whole history of civilisation depends on this trait.
>
> James Williams, 1890

Observation of practice

The apprenticeship model requires supervisors and learners to be together for much of the time. Learning occurs through observing and practising under the observation of the supervisor, who provides appropriate feedback. The usual form of direct observation is where learners and supervisors are together with patients.

Some medical schools use the term *shadowing* to describe what might be almost constant observation by learners of their supervisors. At the postgraduate level, learners usually work independently, spending much less time with their supervisors. Sadly, many supervisors fall into the trap of adopting these pure models. It is easier to have medical students observing than to observe them, and to allow GP registrars to get on with seeing patients, calling in the supervisor as needed. However, at all levels of learning, learners benefit both from observing an experienced clinician in action and from having an experienced clinician observing them with patients. The emphasis might be different, as medical students are able to do less than GP registrars, but sound practice-based teaching uses all three models of sitting in.

Simple observation of supervisors

This is the most commonly used method with medical students. Observation of GPs working through a busy appointment schedule can give learners, particularly those at earlier levels, a reasonable overview of general practice roles and skills. It can also offer learning about the clinical content of the observed consultations, if time is allowed for that. However, too much observation becomes boring for the learner, so it is important to vary the educational menu by allocating other learning tasks to students between sessions of simple sitting in. An interesting variation is to have medical students sitting in with GP registrars. GP registrars often have more free time to talk about each consultation and, as they are in training, should be valuable sources of knowledge. This parallels the hospital-based scenario, where registrars often do more teaching than consultants do. Discussing clinical issues with learners at a lower level is a valuable method of learning.

Simple observation of supervisors also has a valuable role in postgraduate training. It is a useful means of orienting a new registrar to the practice on day one, when the registrar's workload might be light. The registrar could quickly gain an impression of the practice routines and policies and staff roles. The method is also useful beyond day one. Different GPs have different personalities and exhibit different consultation and communication styles. Further, they have different sets of skills and attract different kinds of patients. Hence, even though GP registrars are able to conduct many consultations alone, they will benefit from seeing how others consult. It is a good idea for GP registrars to observe several different general practitioners during training. Group practices have an advantage here, as the observation can be spread around partners and associates.

This form of sitting in is the least disruptive to appointment schedules, depending on how much discussion time is allowed between consultations. A reasonable guide is to schedule four consultations per hour.

Simple observation of learners

Here supervisors sit in with their learners and allow the learner to be largely in control of the consultation. Between consultations, the supervisor provides feedback and a discussion about the case follows. During the consultation the supervisor plays a 'fly- on-the-wall' role, and does not participate in the consultation unless invited to by the learner or to correct a potentially serious error in diagnosis or management. Patients must be aware that they are consulting the learner: this might be difficult with regular patients of the supervisor, as they will tend to talk directly with the supervisor. This model is most commonly used in postgraduate training, where it can lead to interesting discussions around a range of clinical topics, and is the basis of external clinical teaching visits used by the Royal Australian College of General Practitioners (RACGP) training programme. However, it is also valuable with medical students, even if only parts of consultations are observed. For instance, the supervisor might observe the student take a history, conduct an examination or perform a simple practical procedure, but personally conduct the rest of the consultation.

The observation and feedback can be oriented towards consultation skills or particular clinical topics, or both. Consultation skills can be observed in all consultations and this is a good method for their formative assessment, although it lacks the self-assessment capacity offered by videotaping (see next chapter). Feedback could be based on one of the formal rating scales presented in Chapter 4. Much of the interest in this form of sitting in lies in its potential to provide clinical topic tutorials around patient presentations. The learning is highly contextualised to the particular scenario and should be remembered more easily. However, a large number of consultations have to be observed in order to provide clinical teaching on a reasonable number and spread of clinical topics (Hays, 1989), so this is not a particularly efficient form of clinical topic teaching. Strategies for improving the efficiency include arranging the sitting in for selected consultations, such as those with patients with complex, chronic or particular problems. The grounds for selection could be negotiated between supervisor and learner. Clearly, this requires prior planning to ensure that both are free at particular times to see the same patients. Time requirements are usually greater for this form of sitting in; a schedule of three patients per hour is reasonable. An example of how the post-consultation discussion might flow is presented in Box 5.1. Note that the supervisor mostly asks questions and gives direct advice only towards the end, helping the learner to answer their own questions.

In the example, the supervisor did not interrupt the consultation, as agreed before the consultation commenced. However, the consultation should be interrupted if:

- it departs down an incorrect path, with the potential for adverse patient outcomes, in which case the supervisor should intervene (e.g. an incorrect drug is prescribed). This is most unusual
- the learner or supervisor feels that the patient is withholding personal or other information that might be obtained if the observer leaves
- the patient speaks directly with the supervisor. The chance of this can be minimised by placing the observer out of the patient's field of vision.

Box 5.1 An example of how the 'fly-on-the-wall' supervisor (S) might encourage deeper learning after observing a consultation with a learner (L), who in this example is a GP registrar in a basic GP term

Consultation: A 17-year-old female student who presented with an URTI and an anxious mother amid preparation for an important school test tomorrow

S. Well Ahmed, how do you feel that went?

L. Well, I am quite confident that she only had an URTI and so did not need antibiotics, but I felt really pressured by her mother, who more or less demanded some definite course of action. I am not sure that I handled that as well as I should.

S. Precisely what do you think you should have done differently?

L. (pause) Well, I always find it difficult to deal with an anxious parent, but in this case the girl is old enough to speak for herself. I got the impression that the girl would have been happy with advice about paracetamol and a certificate, whereas mum wanted a 'magic bullet' that would fix her by tomorrow morning.

S. At what stage would you feel it reasonable to see adolescents on their own – that is, without a parent?

L. I know what you are getting at – I should have asked the girl to come in alone, but I find that difficult when the parent is just so anxious. Had I done this here, mum might have thought she would not get what she wanted or that we might have spoken about other things.

S. Other things? What sort of things?

L. Sex and contraception, I suppose.

S. Well, that might not be such a bad topic to bring up with a 17-year-old. She might welcome a chance to talk with a doctor as an adult about contraception, relationship problems, STDs etc.

L. But that is really hard to bring up in a consultation about an URTI!

S. Something that I find works well is, after dealing with the URTI, to ask a question like 'What do they teach you about contraception in school?' The answer is usually 'not much', so I then say 'Would you like to ask me any questions about contraception or relationships?' More often than not, the floodgates open, leading to a quite mature information-giving session that could be regarded as useful, opportunistic health promotion. Try it sometime.

L. But you could not do that with mum in the room?

S. Not easily, no. So how would you get mum out of the room?

L. I suppose to just say 'Could I see your daughter alone? She is a big girl now and should be able to give me all the necessary information'.

S. Sounds reasonable. Try it sometime. We had better see the next patient, or you will fall behind.

Conjoint consultations

This form of sitting in is more complex, in that both supervisor and learner participate actively in the consultation. Both might ask questions and conduct parts of the clinical examination, discussing as they proceed. Patients should be aware that they are 'getting two doctors for the price of one', as they could be confused by the three-way conversation. Discussion could continue after the consultation closes.

The commonest application of this method is for consultations involving interesting or complex problems. For example, interesting skin rashes or other visual clues should trigger the calling in by the supervisor of the learner (and vice versa) for an instantaneous joint discussion. Similarly, an ideal way of learning about a particular condition of interest (say, complicated diabetes) is to pre-arrange a conjoint consultation involving a patient with that condition. The supervisor would almost certainly welcome any help the learner can offer! This can be much slower than ordinary consultations; as a rule, allow 30 minutes if a lot of discussion is planned. It is a one-to-one version of the patient-based clinical tutorial used in hospital teaching and is particularly useful for medical student attachments. An example of how a consultation might flow is provided in Box 5.2.

Technical considerations

Consulting rooms are usually designed for one doctor and one or two patients and relatives. Modern architecture and building costs often result in rather cosy rooms with little room for an observer. For the conjoint consultation method this matters less, as both learner and supervisor should be within a comfortable distance and field of vision of the patient. However, for simple observation, the observer should be out of the field of vision of the patient.

This may be difficult to achieve, depending on the size of the room and the location of furniture. The ideal position for the observer is that indicated in Figure 5.1. The observer is at the far apex of a triangle, but is out of the field of vision of both the patient and the person being observed. When this is not possible, the observer should sit as far away from the patient and consulting doctor as possible, keeping quite still and making no sound. If the room design is such that it is impossible to stay out of the field of vision of both patient and doctor, then it is better to stay out of the patient's field of vision.

Box 5.2 Example of a conjoint consultation involving a supervisor (S) and a learner (L), in this case a medical student

The consultation is with a regular attendee, age 71,
with hypertension, diabetes and osteoarthritis

S. Thanks for letting Tania and me see you together today, Mrs Santamaria. Tania and I have just spent a couple of minutes discussing your interesting medical history and now I wonder if you could talk with Tania about why you have come today? I will sit here and just listen for a while – is that OK?

Mrs S. Yes doctor, happy to help.

L. Thank you Mrs Santamaria. So, why have you come today?

Mrs S. This is just my usual check-up.

L. You were last here 1 month ago – how have things been since then?

(The student now takes a history for a couple of minutes, without interruption by the supervisor)

S. So Tania, could you summarise for us all just what is going on with Mrs Santamaria and what we need to do today as a check-up?

L. Mrs Santamaria seems to be managing well with her problems at the moment. Her BSLs are within normal range and she feels well, despite the limitations on activity and diet that she has. She seems to live a fairly active life and to have no new problems at this visit.

S. So what should we do for her today?

L. Check her blood pressure, heart and lungs, her BSL and then give her the prescription.

S. What about her arthritis?

L. Well I suppose we should check all of her joints.

S. Perhaps what we are more interested in is function. Mrs Santamaria has just told you that she has no new problems and that she is fairly active. We also watched her walk in the room a few minutes ago. What did you make of that?

L. It seemed fine.

S. What do you think, Mrs Santamaria?

Mrs S. Yes there is nothing like that worrying me today. It's a chronic thing that gets me down from time to time, but I know that nothing much else can be done.

S. So perhaps that is enough consideration of the osteoarthritis? Would you like to check her blood pressure and chest?

(The consultation continues)

A valuable variant of both forms of simple observation is where the consulting room is fitted with a two-way mirror and adjacent observation room. This is not commonly available in teaching practices. The observer can be truly out of the consultation, yet able to observe, take notes, etc. Several observers can fit into the room, so such facilities are ideal for group learning; hence their value in academic centres. However, it is not as natural as at first glance, because large mirrors, however disguised, look out of place in consulting rooms.

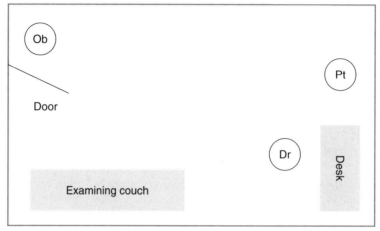

Dr = Doctor, Pt = Patient, Ob = Observer

Figure 5.1 Location of observer for non-participatory sitting in.

Patient consent

Naturally, patients should consent to having a learner in the room with them, particularly if the learner is participating in the consultation. They should know the status of the learner (medical student or postgraduate), understand the role of the learner (just observing or participating) and be aware that they can ask the learner to leave at any time. Ideally, formal written consent should be obtained, similar to that suggested in Chapter 6. However, because the consultation is not recorded, potentially for other uses, a more relaxed approach would be acceptable. It would be advisable to note in the patient record that a learner was present and that the patient consented to this. A convenient way of doing this for written records is to make up a stamp such as that in Figure 5.2. It might also be advisable for the patient to sign underneath the stamp, as that leaves a permanent record of consent. Computerised records could have a word-processor 'macro' with the same information ready to be pulled off a menu and inserted.

DATE:

DOCTOR:

CONSENT: YES ☐
(for learner participation)

Figure 5.2 Suggested stamp for recording patient consent in medical records.

Summary

Observation of supervisors and learners is a very useful learning method that is ideally suited to practice-based teaching. Much of the value is in the timing and relevance of the discussions between learner and supervisor. Learning issues are identified when they occur and in the context of real cases. This has advantages over storing issues to be discussed later, when some details might be forgotten. The method is ideal for formative assessment.

Further reading

Hays RB (1989) The diagnostic content of consultations collected for teaching purposes. *Australian Family Physician.* **1** (7): 846–51.
This paper reports research that shows that, while a valuable teaching and learning strategy, observation of consultations can focus on both process and content of the doctor–patient interaction. However, it requires a substantial number of consultations in order to obtain coverage of more than a restricted range of consultation content.

Hays RB (1990) Content validity of a rating scale for general practice consultations. *Medical Education.* **2** (2): 110–16.
Describes a content-validated, broad general practice rating scale that was developed for Australian general practice.

Hays RB and Peterson L (1996) An evaluation of visiting clinical teachers in general practice teaching. *Education for General Practice.* **7** (1): 54–8.
Results of a study of how sitting in (albeit by visiting teachers) can complement other curriculum delivery.

Neighbour R (1987) *The Inner Consultation.* London: Kluwer Academic Publishers.
A clever approach to consulting more effectively. Neighbour writes well and entertainingly, presenting an unusual approach to monitoring what we do during consultations. His concept of 'safety netting' is very appropriate.

Nyman KC (1996) *Successful Consulting.* Melbourne: Royal Australian College of General Practitioners.
Results of the study of observation of over 2000 consultations, so this is based on rich experience of what GP registrars do during consultations.

Pendleton D and Hasler J (1983) *Doctor–Patient Communication.* London: Academic Press.
Comprehensive coverage of the topic, although quite theoretical in its treatment of common and practical issues. More for those who wish to extend their theoretical understanding.

Pendleton D, Schofield T, Tate P and Havelock P (1984) *The Consultation: an approach to teaching and learning.* Oxford: Oxford University Press.
A practical guide to broadening the assessment of consultations. Written by a team of GPs and a psychologist, this effectively bridges the gap between theory and practice to present a validated framework and rating scale for rating consultations. The scope of the framework is broader than its predecessors, as it includes clinical management as well as communication skills.

Chapter 6

Recording and reviewing consultations

By education most have been misled;
So they believe, because they so were bred.

John Dryden, 1687

Reliving consultations

The step beyond direct observation is the recording of consultations. This can be by either audiotaping or videotaping. Of course, video provides more information, but audiotaping might be sufficient for analysis of history taking and oral communication skills. Both are useful methods for allowing both the supervisor and the learner to replay the consultation at a convenient time. The rationale for reviewing videotaped consultations is that, through self-evaluation and receipt of feedback from others, learners will improve their communication and clinical skills. While this is now more or less standard procedure in general practice training, and can be a powerful tool for analysing the consultation process (Deveugele *et al.*, 2004), recent research has cast some doubt on the strength of improvement in communication skills over time.

One of the reasons for recording consultations is the inherent advantage that learners can get on with work while the microphone or camera quietly records the learner working in the real clinical environment, and therefore it is a form of true performance assessment. Reliving the consultations means that much of the timing and relevance of sitting in (*see* Chapter 5) is maintained, but it adds the capacity for self-observation by learners. However, it requires different techniques and can also provoke some powerful emotions, so participants should be well-prepared or risk not deriving the full benefit. Most of this chapter concerns the use of videotaping, but the principles are similar to those for audiotaping.

Self-confrontation

No matter how brave we are about meeting new people and new situations, humans are not so keen on meeting themselves doing what they normally do. Few people like to hear the sound of their own voice. It usually sounds different to the way we hear ourselves, through a combination of air and bone transmission that others do not detect. Even fewer like to see what we look like to others, as it is often different to the close-ups and angles we see in mirrors. Our mannerisms (yes, we all have them!) seem silly and embarrassing, even though our friends know and accept them as part of us. A video recording can seem quite cruel.

Hence the first step in replaying audiotapes or videotapes of our own consultations is to come to terms with ourselves. Video is the more powerful, as it has more of the auditory and visual information that we need (yet may not want) to observe. Few people find this a comfortable experience. Those with a severe lack of self-confidence often find it very difficult to 'meet' themselves, possibly because of poor self-esteem. The role of the supervisor during debriefing is, therefore, to boost self-image, while ensuring that the learner is aware of what has been done less well.

Here are a few hints for helping learners to get past this awkward stage:

- It helps if supervisors have personally gone through the mental anguish of meeting themselves. This will assist understanding of what their learner is going through. Hard and fast rules are difficult, but supervisors who have not reviewed their own consultations should not expect this of others.
- With all the feeling of experience, supervisors should explain how difficult it can be, but that after a while we get used to ourselves and look at what actually happens in the consultations, at which point the exercise becomes valuable.
- Explore the learner's prior experience with recording of consultations. In some cases it will have been a negative experience, often a group exercise in humiliation conducted poorly by an unaware facilitator. Reassure them that this is a different experience that is for purely personal purposes.
- Allow learners to set up the recording equipment and get used to it, and then turn it on when they feel ready. This may take a few hours or a couple of days.
- Ask learners to review their consultations alone, before sharing them with you. This allows them to feel horrified in private and to get used to hearing and seeing themselves.
- Set up the conjoint review session at a relaxed moment and in a relaxed location, after hours, after a meal, etc.
- Show a videotape of one of your consultations first and invite comment. Following the rules of feedback (*see* Box 6.1), go first and confess your discomfort at hearing and seeing yourself. Also, point out some of the missed cues and arguable issues (there always will be some) in a fairly self-critical (but constructive) way. Ask the learner what he/she would have done differently about specific points of the consultation and value these comments.

Box 6.1 The rules of feedback (modified from Pendleton *et al.*, 1984)

1 Briefly clarify matters of fact
2 The doctor in question goes first
3 Good points first
4 Recommendations, not criticisms
5 Do not leave issues unresolved

- When observing the learner's consultations, follow the rules of feedback closely. Allow the learner to be in control. Be quick to be positive about good points, as the natural tendency is for self-assessors to be overly critical. Focus on the clinical and communication issues that have little to do with the personality and appearance of the learner. It is not necessary to see whole consultations, so allow the learner to select segments to be observed.
- Use the power of questions to facilitate deeper learning. Questions like 'What was going through your mind as you said that?' and 'What did you expect the patient to say in answer to your question?' Focus the discussion on clinical reasoning skills.

- Avoid leaving issues unresolved. That is, if learner and supervisor cannot agree on an issue, one or other (perhaps both should take turns) should agree to research the topic and bring it back for discussion at a future meeting.
- Always acknowledge the learner's progress and contribution to clinical care of the patients concerned. Thank them for the opportunity to get quite close to their thoughts.

Box 6.2 Example of a conversation between a supervisor (S) and a learner (L) during a review of a videotaped consultation. Both have viewed the videotape prior to this conversation

S. Thanks for agreeing to do this, Alfonse. I have been through this too and understand how uncomfortable it can be. You have the remote control and can stop and ask me something, or skip over bits, so long as you can explain why. I will only interrupt to ask questions.

L. Fine, here goes.

(They now start to watch the consultation; after a couple of minutes, the learner stops)

L. I am not sure what you think, but just there I was not sure what to make of that piece of information.

S. At this stage, what did you think was the most likely diagnosis, or diagnoses, that the patient has?

L. Well, the headaches sound like stress headaches to me, but they could be migraine. However, the patient is giving a rather vague history.

S. What do you think the patient is concerned about?

L. Probably something much more serious, like a brain tumour.

S. I think that you were on the right track.

(The videotape continues)

S. Could you just pause for a moment. What was going through your mind when the patient said that?

L. It made me wonder about the psycho-social situation. The patient is not saying so directly, but it appears that there are significant problems at home with the teenage son. I was uncertain about whether to pursue that further at that time or to wait and see what else might come up.

S. You seem to have made a half-hearted attempt to pursue it, then stopped.

L. Yes, but it worked out OK, because the patient went back and continued later to unload a lot of frustration and anxiety.

S. OK, fine.

(The videotape continues, until the learner stops)

L. I really felt out of my depth there. The patient seems to want a referral to yet another neurologist, and is naming a drug that was mentioned as a 'cure' on a television show, but I had never heard of it. I later looked it up and still can't find anything about it.

S. Yes. What do you think the outcome of another referral would be?

L. As this would be the fifth neurology referral, almost certainly nothing new, and perhaps yet another unnecessary set of expensive investigations.

S. How would that help?

L. I don't think it would help much. The patient seems to get temporary relief from another expert reassurance, but then comes back effectively no better.

S. I think that you are correct.

(The tape continues) . . .

There is one important 'don't' in videotape debriefing. Never force a learner to participate beyond their strong discomfort zone. It is fine to gently nudge and cajole, as almost all will find value after the discomfort, but it is possible to further harm those with very low self-esteem by forcing them to meet a person they do not want to meet. Fortunately, very few people are like this.

An example of how to apply this technique with a GP registrar is provided in Box 6.2. The example does not include much clinical context, but demonstrates how a review session allows learners to relive a consultation, reflect on what was said and done, and seek clarification and advice at a time when it would be directly relevant to clinical decision making and, therefore, potentially most useful. The supervisor should ask questions, clarify matters and give supportive advice rather than directly answer questions. Learners often give their own negative feedback and, if not, an appropriate question from the supervisor should focus reflection on an issue that the supervisor wishes to raise.

Technical considerations

Every person who has set up video cameras can tell stories of how, despite careful placement and connecting, the machine did not record, time and effort were wasted, and he or she felt foolish. While it is difficult to guarantee that this will not happen, knowledge of, and experience with, video camera equipment boost the chances of success. There are several different brands and sizes available, so make sure that you are familiar with the one you have. Common traps for the unwary include:

- Check that it is plugged in!
- Check that all the lead plugs are in the right holes.
- Check that the lens cap is off.
- Check that there is a videotape in the machine and that it is rewound.
- Set up the camera at the right angle and distance and press record. Check that it has recorded by replaying the tape through the built-in screen.
- Every so often, check that the 'rec' symbol appears on the screen and that the counter is ticking forward.
- Be alert for the machine automatically and quietly switching to stand-by after a few minutes of 'pause'. There will be a small button somewhere to override this.

This all sounds very simple, but then most errors are.

Advancing technology regularly makes better video cameras available at reasonable cost. Better means smaller and less obtrusive, with better microphone pick-up. The ideal situation is to have two cameras, one focused on the doctor and the other on the patient. This is rarely possible in the real world of general practice, so the next best situation is to have a single camera placed so that it records the body language and facial expressions of both. Sufficient distance is required so that the normal wide-angle range achieves this goal. The best height for the camera lens is about eye-level of a seated person. A suitable arrangement is represented in Figure 6.1.

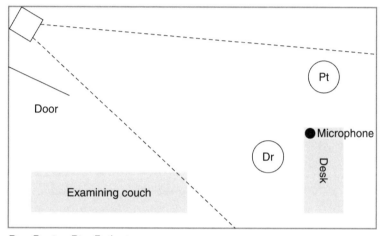

Dr = Doctor, Pt = Patient

Figure 6.1 Recommended arrangement of the video camera in the consulting room.

Consultation room size and design have a major impact. A rectangular room is better, unless the camera has a very wide-angle lens. Extra distance can be gained by attaching the camera to the wall (remember, at about eye-level, sitting, to avoid the impression that observers are looking down on a consultation). A wall fixture also takes up less space and keeps the equipment out of the reach of children, and is a worthwhile investment for practices that regularly have learners. The smaller and less obvious the camera, the better. If funding is available, the best camera to install is a small security camera, as it is an unobtrusive 'eye' wired to controls and recording equipment elsewhere, possibly on a shelf or in an adjacent room.

There is another important 'don't'. The examination of the patient should not be included in the recording. Patient privacy is more important than recording semi-naked bodies. The soundtrack is sufficient to understand what is happening during examinations. If the examination is in an adjacent room, leave the door open so that sound might still be recorded. If the examination is conducted in the consulting room, try to place the camera so that it does not 'see' the couch. If this is not possible, replace the lens cap during the examination. If the examination is too far away to record the sound, then another microphone could be installed in that room.

Microphone sensitivity may also be an issue. Some microphones appear to pick up the sound of cars on the adjacent road better than the voices of two people a few feet away. If this happens, a small, unobtrusive external microphone should be fixed to the desk or a shelf between the doctor and patient. It must be in a position where it cannot be touched during recording, or loud, unwanted noise will come through very clearly. Extraneous noise can be minimised by placing a foam rubber pad between the microphone and the desktop.

Self-evaluation

The most common use of videotape review is to allow for a convenient, private reliving of consultations so that supervisors and learners can provide, receive and discuss feedback about those consultations. In a sense, this is a delayed version of sitting in, with the advantage that learners can see for themselves what they have done well or not so well. It is good for learners to self-assess their performance.

However, one of the real advantages of videotape review is its potential to guide learners in *self-evaluation*. What is the difference? Narrowly defined, evaluation is *measurement against a standard for a purpose*. So self-assessment is a judgement against personal standards and perceptions, while self-evaluation is a judgement against an external standard. If self-directed learners are to base their learning on real needs, then a realistic awareness of their knowledge and skills is better than one that is purely personal.

At the time of reviewing the tapes, an experienced supervisor should be able to make a reasonable judgement regarding the difference between the learner's actual performance and the appropriate level of performance that the learner should have been achieving in the taped consultations. Integrating this external evaluation into the learner's evaluation requires two additional steps, as follows:

- After the learner has observed the consultations, and prior to a conjoint review, the supervisor should observe them alone to make the evaluation.
- After the conjoint review, in which the evaluation is discussed, the learner should observe the consultations again, reflecting on the feedback and discussion.

Ideally, both learner and supervisor should make formal assessments, scoring aspects of the consultations using one of the available rating scales (e.g. Pendleton *et al.*, 1984; Hays, 1990*a*). These rating scales ensure consideration of a wider range of issues involved in consulting, and it takes only a few extra minutes. There is evidence that following this longer procedure produces a more realistic self-awareness of performance in learners (Hays, 1990*b*). There is now at least theoretical support for the importance of the ability to self-evaluate performance throughout a career as a means of developing *insight* into performance and therefore maintaining *currency* of practice (Hays *et al.*, 2002*a*). This provides an additional and important reason to target the raising of self-awareness during training: it may assist the maintenance of future competence.

Consent and security

Consent and security are significant issues when a recording of a consultation is made and kept. Patients could be recognised and their privacy violated if

VIDEO RECORDING CONSENT FORM

Dr . . . . is recording consultations today as part of his/ her training for a higher qualification in general practice. The purpose is to improve his/her skill as a general practitioner. A video camera is situated in one corner of the room so that what you and the doctor discuss will be recorded. The camera will not record any clinical examination for which you might have to undress. You will not be identified by name on the tape.

The recording is strictly confidential and will be kept securely. It will be reviewed only by Dr . . . . and Dr . . . . who is advising on training issues. Once the tape has been reviewed, it will be erased and no-one else can see it. This usually occurs within a few days.

Should you consent to the recording of your consultation, you will be asked to sign the bottom of this form at the end of the consultation. Please note that you may withdraw your consent at any stage during or after the consultation.

Should you not wish your consultation to be recorded, please advise the receptionist now or discuss it with Dr . . . . when you are called in.

— —

I, ..., consent to my consultation with

Dr . . . . on . . . . (date) being video-recorded.

I understand that only Dr . . . . and others involved in general practice training will view it, and that it will be erased within a few days.

. . . .

   Patient Signature   Witness Signature   Date

Figure 6.2 Suggested form of words for video-recording consent leaflet. (Feel free to copy this page and use it in your practice.)

unauthorised persons play the tapes. Formal consent is much more important than for sitting in. An appropriate procedure for gaining informed consent is as follows:

- The receptionist should advise patients on arrival in the practice that the consultation might be recorded. A leaflet explaining the procedure and its purpose should be given to them. After time to digest the material, the receptionist should ask the patients if they have any questions of clarification and check that they agree to the recording. If the patient declines at this stage, the doctor should be advised and should not try to make patients change their minds.
- The doctor should call the patient to the door and, before commencing, check that consent is still given.
- The consultation should proceed. At the end, the doctor should check that the patient is still happy for the recording to be kept and used as specified. The patient should then be asked to sign the consent form.
- The consent form is kept with the patient records.

Some ways of seeking consent are more effective than others. When practice staff and the doctor appear anxious or unhappy about the procedure, their body language and words often transmit the covert, but real, message, and patients often decline.

On the other hand, when the circumstances are explained cheerily like they are a part of normal, modern general practice, and that there are benefits, few patients decline. A draft form of words for consent is shown in Figure 6.2.

An alternative to a separate written consent form is the use of a stamp in the records with similar information to the bottom of the form in Figure 6.2. Computerised record systems could contain a pull-down menu macro for insertion at the appropriate section.

The tapes should be used strictly in accordance with the wording of the consent. Different wording would be required for different purposes. For example, if the consultations might be shown to groups of medical students for a year or two, then the patient must agree specifically to that. Should the consultation be recorded with the form of consent in Figure 6.2, but be regarded as a good one to keep for a broader purpose, then the patient should be contacted and asked to sign a differently worded form of consent. They are unlikely to refuse if asked nicely.

Storage of the tapes should be in a locked cupboard. Patient names should not be visible on the labels.

Other issues

Artificiality

A common complaint about video recording is that the presence of a video camera is unnatural and intimidating. Some find the 'beady black eye' to be an uncomfortable roommate. However, all methods of observation have a similar problem. It is not normal to have another person present in the room, nor does it feel normal to conduct consultations in front of a two-way mirror. The point is that all of these methods are initially discomforting, but the awareness of the slight artificiality soon evaporates as doctor and patient concentrate on the reasons for coming. Video recording is arguably the least intrusive, particularly if a small camera is placed unobtrusively. Learners will often say this after they have got past the self-confrontation. The learner is much more in control and may choose whether or not to show the supervisor particular consultations. However, sitting in and video recording are reasonably interchangeable for much of the desired consultation skills teaching, so it might be appropriate to allow learners to choose which one they prefer.

Sampling

As with sitting in, a large number of recorded consultations need to be observed to ensure that a reasonable range of clinical topics is covered. Hence this method is more suited to the teaching and learning of consulting skills and clinical skills than clinical knowledge, although the latter can be improved through increasing the number of consultations videotaped and arranging for patients with specific problems to come for videotaping. For efficiency, a selection of perhaps three to five consultations should be observed to ensure that a range of issues is covered. This selection could be either random or purposive, based on either what the learner feels is important or the consultation content.

Use in summative assessment

While the most common use of videotaped consultation review is in formative assessment to coach communication and clinical skills, it is possible in both Australia and the UK to choose to submit videotaped consultations for summative assessment. In Australia, candidates in the *Alternative Pathway* and *Performance-based Assessment* routes to Fellowship may choose to collect videotaped consultations instead of sitting the RACGP clinical examination (see www.racgp.org.au for further details). In the UK, candidates for both the JTCGP *Summative Assessment* and the RCGP *Fellowship by Assessment* processes may choose a similar alternative to other clinical assessment methods (see www.jtcgp.org.uk and www.rcgp.org.uk, respectively). There are still some unresolved issues in the summative use, such as whether or not it is possible to set a standard for videotaped consultation review (Hobma *et al.*, 2004), but the method has proven to be valid and reliable (Rethans, 1996; Hays *et al.*, 2002*b*).

Summary

This chapter presents a method for obtaining the maximum benefit from videotape consultation review. Recording of consultations offers many of the advantages of sitting in, together with the ability to review the consultations at a convenient time. This method also offers opportunities for learners to self-assess and, if the correct procedure is followed, to acquire self-evaluation skills and move further towards becoming a self-directed learner. Because consultations can be recorded with little impact on the behaviour of doctor and patient, this offers assessment of actual performance. Correct use of the method requires familiarity with the equipment, the confidence to confront self-images and skilful facilitation. The traditional role is formative assessment, but because of the capacity to assess performance in real clinical practice, review of videotaped consultations is now an option for summative assessment through the alternate pathway and performance assessment routes.

Further reading

Hays RB (1989) The diagnostic content of consultations collected for teaching purposes. *Australian Family Physician.* **1** (7): 846–51.

This paper reports research that shows that, while a valuable teaching and learning strategy, observation of consultations can focus on both process and content, but requires a substantial number of consultations in order to obtain coverage of more than a restricted range of consultation content. The more consultations GP registrars conduct, the broader will be their learning experience.

Hays RB (1990) Content validity of a rating scale for general practice consultations. *Medical Education.* **2** (2): 110–16.

Describes a content-validated, broad general practice rating scale that was developed for Australian general practice.

Hays RB (1990) Self-evaluation of videotaped consultations. *Teaching and Learning in Medicine.* **2** (4): 232–6.

Results of a study that shows that video review can allow learning of more than just consulting skills. With guided self-evaluation from an experienced external observer, learners can achieve deeper learning and improved self-awareness of their performance.

Neighbour R (1987) *The Inner Consultation.* London: Kluwer Academic Publishers.

A clever approach to consulting more effectively. Neighbour writes well and entertainingly, presenting an unusual approach to monitoring what we do during consultations. His concept of 'safety netting' is very appropriate.

Nyman KC (1996) *Successful Consulting.* Melbourne: Royal Australian College of General Practitioners.

Results of the study of observation of over 2000 consultations, so this is based on rich experience of what GP registrars do during consultations.

Pendleton D and Hasler J (1983) *Doctor–Patient Communication.* London: Academic Press.

Comprehensive coverage of the topic, although quite theoretical in its treatment of common and practical issues. More for those who wish to extend their theoretical understanding.

Pendleton D, Schofield T, Tate P and Havelock P (1984) *The Consultation: an approach to teaching and learning.* Oxford: Oxford University Press.

A practical guide to broadening the assessment of consultations. Written by a team of GPs and a psychologist, this effectively bridges the gap between theory and practice to present a validated framework and rating scale for rating consultations. The scope of the framework is broader than its predecessors, as it includes clinical management as well as communication skills.

Chapter 7

Medical record review

> Life is like playing a violin solo in public and learning the instrument
> as one goes along.
>
> Samuel Butler, 1895

The power of the written word

One of the most important roles of a general practitioner is information management. This role includes the maintenance of comprehensive, accurate, meaningful and accessible sets of records that document the healthcare of each patient, and understanding of how this information can improve healthcare management. Where do we learn these skills? Not from lectures, but from observing and participating in good information management. This should be regarded as a clinical skill, which could be learned during practice attachments. Whereas medical students should grasp the principles, postgraduate learners should become proficient.

This chapter will focus on the review of patient records and other commonly stored information for educational purposes, rather than the technology, which is a substantial topic on its own. Patient records have a powerful educational role, as they document the clinical findings, thoughts and reasoning of the writer. Reviewing patient records provides a kind of reliving of consultations, with the advantage that their serial nature can makes cases unfold in a relatively short period of time. Teaching and learning involving patient records have two distinct roles: to foster development of good information management skills, and as a medium for clinical teaching.

Good record keeping

An overview of what constitutes good record keeping is a useful prerequisite to the educational discussion. The purpose of patient records is to provide a meaningful record of the healthcare of each patient. This has two elements – information and meaning. Recording information is relatively easy, so long as there is space. General practice records should contain the following information:

- demographic information, such as age, gender, address, occupation, etc.
- a healthcare summary, including: past medical history; family history; current problems; medication lists; allergies; vaccinations; use of tobacco, alcohol and other drugs; and social/family issues. A current healthcare summary is a cornerstone of sound medical practice
- continuation notes, with an entry for each clinical encounter, whether in the surgery, at home or by phone
- results of investigations
- correspondence, both in and out. This includes copies of referral letters sent and reports received.

These requirements are equally relevant for paper-based and computerised systems. Computerised information management systems are improving continually, so the need for large paper storage areas might reduce in the near future, although many challenge the idea that a totally paperless system will be possible. Computers fit much more into a small space, but need back-up systems as they can 'crash'. However, as faster operating systems develop and doctors become more computer-wise, more practices will adopt the technology.

The second feature of good patient records – meaningfulness – is equally important. It is not much use having masses of information that does not mean much. Meaning is required for several purposes, as follows:

- The content must mean something to the doctor who contributes to the records. The provision of continuing care requires a meaningful, ongoing record that tells a story. This is the easiest level of meaning, because we often develop a personal form of shorthand and cryptic symbols that summarise our findings and thoughts.
- The content must have meaning to other health professionals. Increasingly, patients see more than one GP and others in the healthcare team. Continuing, comprehensive care now requires that records have meaning that can be understood by those other than the individual doctor who sees the patient. This means that personal shorthand and cryptic symbols are not a good idea (unless the practice has a common set) and that legibility is essential. In a sense, any experienced GP should be able to make meaning of the record, should they be consulted by the patient in your absence.
- The content must have meaning for other groups. Increasingly, individuals and organisations outside of the practice have access to patient records. The patient themselves, through their legal adviser, the courts and regulatory authorities can all obtain access for specific purposes. Insurance companies, with patient permission, can ask for reports of past presentations. Meaning, in a medicolegal sense, requires that the doctor's actions are clearly understandable, so that they can be compared with peer expectations. Difficulties often arise because records are insufficiently detailed to allow for a clear understanding of the clinical findings and clinical reasoning at the time.

However, a word of caution is in order. Any interpretation of patient records must acknowledge the fact that they are unlikely to represent exactly what happened. There is evidence from the Netherlands that what GPs write in their records is often different to what they actually do during the consultations. This was based on a study which videotaped consultations and then analysed the patient records (Rethans *et al.*, 1994). This situation is probably universal, as a written record is only an abstraction of a complex interaction.

Referral letters and other correspondence

Writing referral letters is another skill that is poorly taught, but easily learned. Good referral letters are typed on practice letterhead and contain the following information:

- age, gender, address and other identifying information of the patient being referred

- the reason for the referral (advice, take over management, procedure, etc.)
- a brief history of the presenting complaint
- relevant background (current problems, past medical history, family history, social and occupational history, etc.)
- the diagnostic impressions of the referring doctor
- a list of current medications
- the desired future role of the referring doctor.

There may also be correspondence with other general practices, insurance companies, solicitors, etc.; all have educational potential.

Computerised records

Most general practice medical records are now computerised. This means that poor legibility is now unusual and completed patient records are comprehensive, accessible, informative and helpful. However, GPs may have poor typing skills and 'makw many spelling anf grammatical; errors', it may not be possible to store all material (referral letters, reports and images take up a lot of electronic space) and busy GPs often do not complete all sections. Further, as anyone who has lived through a computer system crash would know, when the system is down (they all crash occasionally) the practice almost ceases to function.

Fortunately, regardless of format (paper-based or electronic), the principles of good record keeping are the same, with the addition of IT security (confidentiality and back-up procedures), as are the principles for their use as a learning tool.

Learning good record keeping

This is a clinical skill and it should be learned in much the same way as other clinical skills. Learners should observe good record keeping in the practice records, they should discuss record keeping with their supervisor, and they should receive feedback at regular intervals about the content and meaning of their own contributions. This is usually easy to arrange, as supervisors and learners often see the same patients, even in advanced stages of postgraduate training.

Medical students should also contribute to patient records where they contribute to consultations. They are likely to want to write more content than experienced doctors, more as an independent essay than as a chapter in a longitudinal healthcare story, but to do this is an important stage of learning. It is probable that, for longer-term meaning, the most appropriate amount of information to record is somewhere between what the learner and the 'old hand' would write. Perhaps they could learn from each other?

Clinical teaching with patient records

Patient records are a written recording of what took place during consultations. Although they do not provide verbatim transcripts, let alone sound of conversations and picture of actions, they can provide a valuable window on the clinical method of the writer, as well as topics for case-based clinical teaching. Any part of the record, including referral letters and results, can be useful learning triggers. Some suggestions are listed in Box 7.1.

Box 7.1 Clinical documentation with potential teaching value

- Patient records
- Referral letters
- Test results
- Work certificates
- Death certificates
- Applications for nursing home places
- Letters to solicitors, insurance companies and other third parties

---

Setting up record review

This is an activity that can fit easily into a discussion over a coffee or meal break, although a formal teaching appointment would be better. At the practice and within practice hours is best, because the records are kept at the practice.

Which patient records?

Reviewing all records written by learners is unrealistic, so a method of sampling is required. There are two methods, as follows:

- Purposive sampling, or selecting patient records that meet particular criteria. These might be records of patients who are particularly challenging, have a particular condition (e.g. diabetes), have thick files, were seen in particular contexts (home visits or nursing homes), or were seen previously. This is a good method for tailoring clinical teaching to learning needs identified by other means.
- Random sampling. Strategies include asking a receptionist to retrieve 'all records of patients seen this morning' or last Wednesday, or on any other occasion. Perhaps only every third or fourth record will then be reviewed, due to time constraints. This is an appropriate method, discussing 'generic' clinical method issues, for reassuring the learner that their content knowledge is developing and for identifying new learning needs.

Reviewing the patient record

The rules of engagement are similar to those for most forms of clinical teaching and follow the usual feedback rules. Supervisors should demonstrate the method by asking the learner to review one of his or her patient records. Steps are as follows:

- The learner reads through the record and is given an opportunity to comment first on the consultation. As with other forms of self-confrontation, some comments will be critical.

- The supervisor asks questions of clarification. Such questions as 'What was going through your mind as you wrote that bit?' are useful ways of exploring the clinical reasoning.
- Feedback should include positive comments, such as, 'Oh yes, I see what you mean', or 'Yes, that is what I would have thought'.
- Supervisors should raise concerns through comments or questions, rather than direct criticisms.
- Play 'hypotheticals', by using the patient record to explore broader issues. Questions like, 'What if the patient had had an enlarged liver?', 'What would you expect to see at the next consultation?', 'What do you think the results of those tests will be?' or 'What if the result comes back tomorrow abnormal?'.
- The supervisor asks the learner if he or she would do anything differently next time.
- End with acknowledgement of the learner's contribution and thanks for discussing personal thoughts.

A North American term for using patient records to explore clinical knowledge is 'chart stimulated recall'. This is a very powerful learning tool, as it allows for more elaborated contextual learning about not just the particular case being discussed, but a range of similar cases that feel quite real. It comes close to replicating, in discussion format, the clinical reasoning process of learners. The original thought that it might be a method of 'teaching' clinical reasoning is no longer held, but it is still regarded as a useful method of clinical teaching, because it allows exploration of 'what if' scenarios that can cover a wide range of clinical possibilities. It is also becoming more popular as an assessment tool, usually formative, often known as a 'case-based oral'.

Summary

This chapter has presented a framework for using patient records as a powerful tool in practice-based clinical teaching and assessment. The methods should be relevant regardless of the format of records. The chart-stimulated recall method is also used as a summative assessment tool in some settings because of its capacity to assess performance in a range of actual clinical cases.

Further reading

Del Mar C, Lowe JB, Adkins PB and Arnold E (1996) What is the quality of general practice records in Australia? *Australian Family Physician (REASON)*. **25**: S21–5.
  Results of research into what records should contain and how their quality can be measured. One result is a validated patient record rating scale that has been shown to measure improvement in quality of record keeping.
Royal Australian College of General Practitioners (2005) *Standards for General Practice* (3e). Sydney: RACGP.
  Includes, among many issues for which standards can be defined and measured, one approach to defining what medical information systems should contain and how they should be used.

Chapter 8

Making the most of one-to-one tutorials

> Men [and women] learn while they teach.
>
> Seneca, c.4 BC – c. AD 65
> (additional words added by the author!)

Formal, flexible and fun

Educational organisations often provide a list of topics that should be covered by learners during a practice attachment. Sometimes they require that the supervisor and learner spend formal structured teaching time together. This is often poorly done, partly because of time pressure, but partly because one-to-one tutorials that follow a list of topics can be rather uninteresting for both participants and not particularly valuable for the learner. Chapters 5, 6 and 7 have shown that topics will emerge from sitting in, audio/video review and medical record review. This chapter discusses how other strategies can make structured teaching time both more enjoyable and more powerful learning experiences.

Why have tutorials?

The main roles of structured teaching time are to augment experiential learning from seeing patients and to ensure coverage of required curriculum content. The list of topics provided by the educational organisation is indicative of the clinical content areas that learners are expected to learn about during the attachment and should reflect learning objectives, but should not necessarily be seen as a list of tutorial topics. Instead, the ongoing monitoring of progress towards achievement of the learning goals should identify what has been achieved through experiential learning (seeing patients and exploring issues concerning their problems) and what has so far not been achieved. Experiential learning is rather opportunistic, in that the 'curriculum comes in through the door', but there is no guarantee that the patients encountered in a particular attachment will reflect all of the required topics. Should a particular topic not be adequately covered, the supervisor and learner should then arrange a time, a place and a strategy – a kind of one-to-one tutorial – for achieving this.

Hence these tutorials are a very important aspect of clinical supervision. As with other supervision methods, this one requires careful planning and implementation in order to optimise its value. As with all teaching time, tutorials should be scheduled and kept free of telephone calls, paperwork and consultations, except in an emergency. Several teaching and learning strategies are ideal for these sessions; these are listed in Box 8.1 and discussed further below. As each topic is covered and each learning objective is achieved, they can be checked off on the list of required topics. The need for these tutorials might become greater towards the end of the attachment, should there be several outstanding topics not covered through experience and opportunism.

Box 8.1 Teaching and learning strategies ideal for structured teaching time

- Critical incident analysis
- Critical appraisal
- Arranged consultations
- Simulated consultations

A universal requirement for all of these tutorial methods is to engage the learner and to hand over responsibility for learning. This means not giving direct answers to learners' questions, but rather using the power of questioning to enhance deeper learning. One effective strategy is to answer each question with another, reflecting the question back to the person, who should know how to find the answer. For example, if asked 'What is the best drug to use in hyperlipidaemia?', the supervisor should respond with 'How would you find that out?' Where possible, guide the learner to solve his or her own problems, using whatever educational resources are available. In a sense, here the learner becomes the teacher, not only of him or herself, but also of the supervisory teacher.

Critical incident analysis

Critical incident analysis is a form of quality assurance activity that originated in the military forces as a means of learning from errors. Military errors are often high-stakes events that cost lives and see expensive equipment lost. Incorrect judgements or decisions made by humans are often the cause of the adverse outcome (e.g. 'pilot error' in an aircraft crash). However, incidents often follow a chain of decisions, each of which depends on a prior decision. Therefore, *post hoc* analysis of an adverse event may lead to an improved understanding of what went wrong and why things went wrong. The emphasis is on avoiding repetition of the error, rather than apportioning blame to individuals. This can be a powerful learning tool.

Many errors in medical practice are similar, in that patient outcomes are affected by decision pathways that have many steps, each of which affects the next. Humans make most decisions, so humans make most of the errors, although some are due to equipment failures or incorrect results. Quite serious adverse outcomes can also result.

The first medical practitioners to adopt a critical incident approach were anaesthetists, for whom adverse outcomes are uncommon, but often tragic. However, the approach is also relevant to general practitioners, even though we are not usually making high-stakes decisions that mean a difference between life and death. The same method can also be applied to pathways with good outcomes, because identifying how and why good outcomes occur is also a useful learning opportunity. The method is particularly relevant to vocational training, rather than medical school education, as GP registrars are more independent and more responsible for direct patient care. This chapter explains how critical incident analyses can be applied in the context of practice-based supervision.

Critical incidents in general practice

An example of an error in clinical decision making in general practice is shown in Figure 8.1. The difficult issue of detecting (or not detecting) a tumour at a stage when the prognosis could be improved is depicted by a series of steps. This is of course a gross simplification, as it is difficult to include all of the information on which a decision to investigate, or not to investigate, is made. This includes: duration of symptoms, nature of the bleeding, family history, weight loss, etc., and an assessment of the haemorrhoids and the risk of dual pathology.

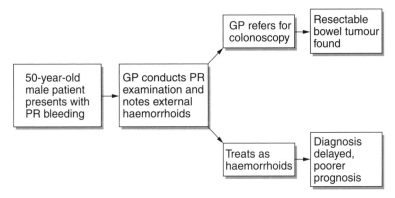

Figure 8.1 An example of a critical incident pathway analysis with a poor outcome.

Hence, from the point of view of the GP, the most important steps to analyse are the first two (that is, history taking and examination). There could be a number of reasons why the GP chose not to investigate further at that stage, such as: the patient not revealing all of the relevant history; or the GP not listening to, or not seeking, the relevant history. Even if the GP had referred the patient for a colonoscopy, the patient might not have attended, with a similar result. Investigating exactly what happened along this clinical pathway should be a useful, if painful, reflection on actual practice. It is therefore a valuable learning experience, particularly if the individual concerned seeks the evidence and personally identifies the critical steps where the pathway deviated.

Critical incident analysis in general practice training

The best description of critical incidents in general practice training comes from a Western Australian study (Diamond *et al.*, 1995). This study collected information on 180 incidents recorded by 39 GP registrars during their first (basic) general practice attachments (six months' duration). Close to half of all incidents were reported as having positive outcomes. Interestingly, communication and counselling skills were identified as being the important step in the pathways, whether positive or negative. While this study was a research project rather than an educational intervention, it provides a sound basis for developing educational strategies for employing the method routinely. Errors of judgement occur commonly enough, so it is likely that the supervisor, the learner or both will make errors of judgement during longer attachments. This 'critical incident' should be used as the basis of a one-to-one topic tutorial, regardless of the topic concerned. The key issue is often about clinical decision making – a process issue, but required topics often include process of care issues – and there is usually a worthwhile 'moral' to be learned. It also allows a required topic to be mentally marked off as having been achieved.

Rules for conducting such a session are shown in Box 8.2. Critical incidents are rather personal events that sometimes stir strong emotions, particularly if the 'owner' believes that he or she is personally responsible for an adverse outcome. The principles of providing feedback should be followed, by being supportive and treating the information as confidential. The 'owner' of the case should be in the chair and should be encouraged to identify the 'moral' to the story, or 'what I should (or should not) do next time'. An example is 'When I am on call after hours I will always seek the advice of my supervisor when I am not sure what to do'. Supervisors should role-model the appropriate professional behaviour by presenting their own cases from time to time, particularly positive cases, and demonstrating that they, too, have something to learn. The model is also ideal for small groups of learners; this is discussed more in Chapter 9.

Box 8.2 Rules of engagement for critical incident discussions

1 The supervisor should role-model by presenting one of his/her own critical incidents.
2 Only the 'owner' of the critical incident should make negative comments about it.
3 The listener should briefly clarify matters of fact.
4 Discussion should be non-judgemental.
5 The listener should be supportive when negative comments are made.
6 Presentation of positive cases should be encouraged.
7 Both participants should attempt to identify a 'moral' to the story.
8 The main object is to learn from the incident.
9 The cases and discussions are confidential to the participants.

The usual result of using the critical analysis strategy is relief on the part of the 'owner' of a problem. The critical incidents usually fall into categories, such as those identified in the research paper: interpersonal skills, diagnostic skills, management skills and attitudes. Most critical incidents are presented as if they have not happened before, whereas of course they have, particularly to the supervisor, and probably to some of the registrar's peers. Just knowing that this is not the only incident of its kind is helpful. Once the relief sets in, participants are freed to look for learning points and 'morals'.

Critical appraisal

Critical appraisal is the ability to interpret information and is the basic tool of evidence-based medicine (EBM). In the usual academic context, it is often interpreted as the ability to make sense of research papers, or to ensure that their claims are based on sound methods and interpretations of relevance to clinical practice. Most learners will have received ample tuition in this more formal critical appraisal, so supervisors should also be familiar with it. The *British Medical Journal* (*BMJ*) series on 'How to Read a Paper' is worth reading (Greenhalgh, 1997a–d).

Critical appraisal in general practice can be a little different. GPs will not often search original research literature, instead relying on abstracting services that (we trust) perform the critical appraisal for us. However, when GPs do access research literature, there are sound principles to follow. First, if time is short, read only those clinical research papers that address a question that is meaningful to the general practice. That is, the question should relate to clinical issues that are encountered in general practice. Second, the research should be conducted in a general practice setting, with patients that are likely to be seen in general practice. As an example, a study of the effectiveness of antibiotics for acute sore throat should collect data in a general practice or primary care setting from patients that are commonly seen by GPs. Third, the correct methods should be applied in the design. For example, a blinded randomised clinical trial is the most effective design for answering which intervention is best, but is often not feasible in a general practice context. Fourth, the analysis (often statistical methods) must be appropriate to the design and the data collected. Finally, the interpretation of data and suggested application should make sense to GPs. These issues are summarised in Box 8.3.

For a deeper understanding of these issues, see *Evidence-based Medicine* (Sackett *et al.* 1997) and *Evidence-based Practice in Primary Care* (Silagy and Haines, 1998).

Box 8.3 Critical appraisal issues for general practitioners

- Is the research question relevant to general practice?
- Does the setting of the research reflect general practice/primary care?
- Are the methods appropriate to the question and the setting?
- Is the data analysis appropriate?
- Does the interpretation reflect the data collected and analysed?
- Do the conclusions appear to be meaningful to general practice?

Critical appraisal as a tutorial strategy

So far, critical appraisal might not sound like an appropriate ingredient for a practice-based one-to-one tutorial. However, it depends on how it is used. A discussion of the merits and relevance of a recent paper to a particular patient or clinical topic is a powerful tool. Here the discussion is less about the research design and more about relevance to the discipline of general practice, and often a specific patient that is currently being seen by the learner.

It is useful to keep a collection of papers that address clinical content areas that are on the required list and/or are current topical issues. Ideally, some should be meta-analyses, or summaries of pooled data from combining similar studies. Examples are listed in Box 8.4. All of these are common general practice issues that are likely to be encountered by a learner during a practice attachment. A method for using them is illustrated in Figure 8.2.

Box 8.4 Recent papers on topics such as these are worth keeping for teaching purposes

- The effects of raised lipid levels and of lipid lowering agents
- Comparisons of common and new anti-hypotensive agents
- The early detection of, and intervention for, prostate cancer
- Comparisons of common and new anti-asthma drugs
- Comparisons of treatments for impotence

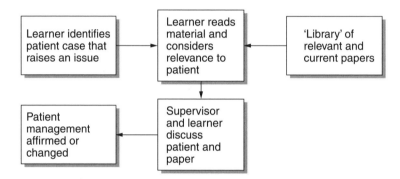

Figure 8.2 Use of critical appraisal of information relevant to clinical cases.

This section has so far dealt with more traditional sources of information. However, more common sources of new information for GPs include pharmaceutical company representatives, Health Departments, the National Health and Medical Research Council, special interest groups and medical newsletters. Most weeks, GPs are bombarded with a wide range of information from many sources and presenting information of variable quality.

Hence critical appraisal in practice should reflect this diversity, variability and the need to develop ways of managing information overload. The method in Figure 8.2 could be followed, but the information used could be drawn from any source, such as pharmaceutical company marketing material or an internet website. Critical appraisal may not indicate that all such material is necessarily of inferior quality, but will show it is certainly of variable quality. Learners need to learn to see through the ploys to attract the attention of readers, such as colour, pictures, famous names, selective quoting and rewards.

Arranged consultations

Because practice-based learning is partly opportunistic and random, based on what comes through the door, patients illustrating some of the required curriculum content might not come through that door during a particular attachment. Learners are transients in the practice, so they usually have most involvement with those patients who do not mind seeing another practitioner.

This includes those with relatively acute problems that could be cared for by other than their usual GP, such as URTIs. Hence the 'through the door' curriculum for learners is often biased towards the simpler and more acute conditions, for which continuity of care is less of a concern. Getting around this narrow exposure requires the supervisor to improvise, although preferably in a way that provides clinical experience, rather than falls back on a more didactic method.

All supervisors and practices should have patients that illustrate all required curriculum issues (otherwise the curriculum does not reflect actual practice!). Hence, should a gap be recognised during the regular progress review sessions, the supervisor should arrange for a patient with the required characteristics to attend for a consultation with the learner, preferably alone. Most such patients, when asked, will accept seeing a different doctor for a special occasion, particularly if the regular doctor explains why and sees them at the end of the consultation. The encounter is an ideal vehicle for a one-to-one tutorial on the clinical topic involved and on the nature of continuing, comprehensive care.

The most appropriate 'arranged' consultations are often those with patients who have chronic illnesses that are best managed in a continuing relationship. Examples include diabetes, asthma and ischaemic heart disease. While this strategy does not involve long-term follow-up of the patient and true responsibility by the learner personally, the learner still becomes involved in real management discussions for topics that are required by the curriculum. Longer attachments provide opportunities for the learner to participate in several 'arranged' consultations, thus providing the potential for a degree of continuing, comprehensive involvement.

Simulated consultations

Sometimes, learning might be reinforced through discussion of patients other than those who have been seen, either opportunistically or in an arranged manner. The more often a learner works through cases on similar topics, the more likely it is that the information and the approach will be stored in contextual knowledge, from which it can be retrieved more easily. One way of achieving this is to work through simulated cases that represent the required curriculum topics.

While many quite sophisticated simulations exist in academic centres, practice supervisors will have to use much simpler ones such as written cases (e.g. cases described in journals) and cases from their memories. Remembered cases are particularly valuable, as they are based on real patients and often have a 'moral' in the tale. Presenting cases that highlight genuine challenges, rather than personal triumphs, are usually more valuable. Again, supervisors should keep a file of interesting cases (written or 'real') that cover interesting and required topics. Learners, too, may be able to remember past cases that raise the same, or similar, issues. Reworking these can be a valuable learning experience.

One powerful method is for the supervisor or the learner to role-play one of their memories. Here the focus is less on communication skills and more on the clinical content, and the method may be combined with critical appraisal of written material to ensure deeper learning around the case. Even without a real patient, learners can work through consultation scenarios and learn from them.

With experience, this can happen quickly, thus compressing several patient simulation discussions into a relatively short period of time.

Summary

This chapter has presented some methods of making topic tutorials more interesting and adult learning oriented. Ideally, few such tutorials will be necessary, as the clinical experience should be broad enough to allow learners to experience first hand the required range of curriculum topics. When this does not happen, or when further discussion is required, particularly for an exploration of an evidence base for management decisions, then these methods should help supervisors plug curriculum gaps in a way that is still active learning linked to actual practice experience.

Further reading

British Medical Journal series 'How to Read a Paper'. *BMJ,* vol. 315, 1997. For example:
    Greenhalgh T (1997) How to read a paper: assessing the methodological quality of published papers. *BMJ.* **315**: 305–8.
    Greenhalgh T (1997) How to read a paper: getting your bearings (deciding what the paper is about). *British Medical Journal.* **315**: 243–6.
    Two of a series that covers most aspects of critical appraisal in a brief and easy-to-read format.
Diamond MR, Kamien M, Sim MB and Davis J (1995) A critical incident study of general practice trainees in their basic general practice term. *Medical Journal of Australia.* **162**: 321–4.
    The paper that best explains how critical incident analysis can guide general practice training.
Sackett D, Richardson WS, Rosenberg W and Haynes RB (1997) *Evidence-based Medicine.* London: Pearson Professional Publishing.
    Comprehensive coverage of applying EBM in an educational framework, albeit in a hospital-oriented setting.
Silagy C and Haines A (eds) (1998) *Evidence-based Practice in Primary Care.* London: BMJ Books.
    The most current and comprehensive book on this topic. It includes some excellent practical advice on 'how to', along with theory and methods.

Chapter 9

Small group practice-based supervision

> Teaching medical students in a teaching hospital is like trying to teach forestry in a lumber yard.
>
> Anon

A broader role for practice-based learning

As mentioned in Chapter 1, educational organisations are changing the way they teach clinical subjects, particularly at medical school level. Teaching hospitals are increasingly unlikely to offer students the range of clinical problems they need to know about, because of increasing high-technology specialisation of their case-load. Except for specialised postgraduate topics, learners are more likely to achieve competence by encountering and learning from those patients with the common and ordinary problems that general practitioners must master.

Hence there is a trend towards placing more learners in community-based clinical practices, for longer attachments. In addition, as healthcare systems move further towards community-based care delivery, this trend will accelerate. Although the traditional model of attaching learners to community practices sees the apprenticeship of one learner to one supervisor, there is no reason why this cannot be extended to include small group patient-based teaching, just as occurs in traditional hospital contexts. Indeed, resource constraints mean that small group teaching is more efficient. Whilst this is unlikely to replace those parts of subjects that are better delivered through centralised lectures and skills laboratories, it should be seen as complementary to other forms of learning. Community-based supervisors will simply do more of the practical supervision.

This form of practice-based teaching is different to the traditional one-to-one model presented in other chapters. An adult learning approach is still the most appropriate, but this approach can be extended to encourage groups of students to become the focus, the engine and the monitor of learning. Supervisors need not spend more time on the educational tasks to achieve this, but rather use their time differently, so that the group process empowers group members to achieve their learning objectives. This can be a lot of fun. This chapter shows how, using examples drawn from both medical student and vocational training contexts.

Group dynamics

Groups comprise individuals, each of whom has a different personality, attitude, level of interest and, perhaps, learning style. The secret of facilitating small group learning is to get the group working together in an environment of mutual trust on a common task. Several factors may have an impact on this.

The first factor is group size. The ideal group comprises six to eight learners. Fewer than six reduces the interactivity, more than eight increases the risk of leaving some members out of the action. Community-based supervisors are very unlikely to have large groups of students, so this section will focus on dealing with small groups, perhaps as few as two. Furthermore, group members might be attached to a number of adjacent practices, so the group process might have to survive periods of physical separation. The smaller the number of learners in the group, the nearer the model of supervision approaches that suggested for a sole learner. That is, with two learners, supervisors could behave much the same way as with a sole learner, although they can get the learners to work together on some tasks.

The second factor is the nature of individual members, although a skilled facilitator can get most groups working together. Supervisors will have little or no choice over who is in their group, and so will have to work with whoever they are sent. Further, it is quite possible that the group members will also not know each other prior to meeting with the supervisor. It is important to get to know a little about each learner and for each learner to get to know each other learner and the supervisor, quite early in the attachment. The long way to do this is to have an education meeting with each group member. This is a good idea with smaller numbers (two to three), but increasingly impractical with larger numbers. This approach also does not help learners get to know each other.

The most efficient way is to commence with a group meeting. The supervisor introduces him or herself, briefly providing sufficient details of his or her clinical and professional life to allow the learners to understand what an attachment in this community can offer. The supervisor should include some personal information, because it is important for learners to learn how practitioners function as individuals within families and communities. Each group member is then asked to introduce him or herself and say what they hope to get out of the attachment. An example introduction for a rural supervisor hosting a group of medical students is suggested in Box 9.1.

Box 9.1 A sample introductory comment

Hello everybody. My name is Susan Johnson and my role here in [name of community] is to make sure that you learn a lot from your time here and that you enjoy your stay. I have been a general practitioner for six years and have worked part-time for the university for two years.

This is a small group practice of three doctors and we work closely with the local hospital and the other four practices in the surrounding communities. During your stay, each of you will be attached mainly to one practice, but you will spend time in each of the practices and in the hospital. You will spend time with our resident physiotherapist and social worker, and with the visiting surgeon and physician when they are here. We also have a really supportive community and local people will take you under their wing and show you what it is like to live in a country town.

I am married and have three children at pre-school and primary school. You will meet all of them at a barbecue this weekend. I really enjoy my work here and I hope that by the end of your attachment, you will understand what it is like to be a rural GP.

Now that I have told you a little about myself, I would like each of you to introduce yourself and to say what you hope to get out of this attachment.

A third factor is the skill of the facilitator (supervisor). Just as one-to-one supervision aims to empower individuals to learn from their attachment, the aim of small group supervision is to empower a group learning experience which enables individuals to learn. More will be said of this later.

A model of small group supervision

This section will simply point out the modifications to the model presented in Chapter 2, as principles of adult learning and supervision apply as much in the small group context as they do with individuals. A summary of the principles of supervising small groups is provided in Box 9.2.

Box 9.2 Principles of small group process

- Plan group processes carefully
- Regularly review process
- Separate chairing and facilitation roles
- Maintain participation of all members
- Allow group to elect chairpersons and allocate tasks
- Encourage group members to find answers to their questions
- Encourage frequent feedback to participants
- Include a variety of educational strategies, as suggested by the content

---

Educational planning is still essential and should involve the whole group. The introduction suggested in Box 9.1 begins this process by asking each learner to explain what he or she hopes to get out of the attachment. It is likely that, when combined, the list of expectations will be substantial and varied. It is useful to have these written on a whiteboard and have the group work out which ones are the most important. The course objectives are also a useful contribution, but individual learners may choose to learn in greater depth or breadth. So long as the course objectives are covered, this is to be facilitated. Allow the group to allocate learning objectives to each other, such that each learner will have an opportunity to explore particular objectives in greater depth. Group learning has the potential to 'unlock' opportunities for individuals to pursue different learning objectives and contribute what they learn to group discussions. By the end of this first meeting, each member (including the facilitator) should have a clear idea of where and how to proceed.

Regular review of progress is still essential, particularly for longer attachments; this can be done rapidly. In between meetings, learners will pursue their learning objectives and should meet to share what they have gained. At least once per week, the facilitator should join in and formally review progress, amending objectives or arranging learning opportunities as indicated.

Feedback should be provided to group members as necessary, but modified rules are required. First, it is more difficult to give negative feedback to individuals in a group situation than alone. It is probably better not to try, but rather make arrangements to talk with the individual alone later. Second, feedback is often better given by the group, just as individual feedback is often better given as self-assessment. Group members will know each other better than will the facilitator, and should be able to make their views known in a supportive way. Groups that work well can often do this very openly and without attacking egos. The main role of the facilitator is to ensure that other members do not harass 'weak' group members. In a sense, group function is in the hands of all members. More about feedback skills is provided later.

Group tutorials are a useful way of imparting the supervisor's distilled clinical experience to a group of learners. There are times when a burst of didactic teaching can be helpful, particularly for topics that are not well covered in textbooks or journals and for practical skills. However, there are a few rules:

- Be brief and precise, or risk boring people.
- Be practical, as that is your expertise. Theory is often better explained elsewhere.
- Where possible, demonstrate rather than just talk. If possible, provide opportunities for practical skills to be practised and feedback provided.
- Always check that your message has been understood.
- Do not try to answer all the questions asked of you.

Similarly, small groups can be vehicles for other specific teaching and learning strategies, such as 'games' (e.g. debates), breaking into pairs, practical skills sessions, etc. Small group learning is not so much a strategy in itself as a medium in which to apply other educational strategies.

Group facilitation 'micro-skills'

There is a set of facilitator behaviours that optimise learning opportunities for individual group members. In combination, they might produce an appearance of passivity in the facilitator, when they are really very active. These are not difficult to master, although they require thoughtful control of relatively natural responses.

'Say little, think hard' sums up the 'invisible control' aspect of the facilitation role. Facilitators are there to guide, rather than direct, learners. Good groups do most of this for themselves. It is important to watch and listen very carefully to group interactions and to intervene only when invited to by the group or if the group appears to be going too far down the wrong direction. Even so, be careful not to give away too much, as it is normal (even productive) for learners to feel a bit lost or to go down a blind alley every so often. After all, that sounds just like healthcare practice! Speaking should be restricted to getting the group going, responding to questions from the group, redirecting groups which are thoroughly lost and ensuring that quieter members have a say. It is quite difficult to perform this kind of 'active listening' role.

There is a difference between facilitating and chairing. This is really a strategy for achieving the 'say little, think hard' role. The chairing role is an administrative and organisational role to ensure that the business items of a meeting are dealt with, whereas facilitation requires much more than this, as it ensures that the learning process is appropriate, both for the group as a whole and for each individual member. A useful strategy is to arrange for one of the learners to chair the meeting, as this frees you to observe and guide the learning process.

Questioning is a powerful tool. Learners often look to the facilitator for an answer, and the facilitator probably knows one that is reasonable. However, avoid giving answers too easily. Instead, reflect the question back to the group, perhaps reframing it in a way that allows members to see how to get the answer for themselves. This promotes a higher level of learning. An important part of learning is knowing how and where to get an answer, rather than being spoon-fed. This is a difficult skill for facilitators to develop, as the natural and quick response is to comply. Naturally, providing an answer might be appropriate in certain circumstances, such as when an answer to part of the question leads the learners in the right direction to discover the rest of the answer, so try to avoid frustrating learners by leaving them uncertain about what to do next.

Flexibility is necessary, as different responses are needed for different situations. The role of tutorial-giver appears to conflict with the previous section, but it need not, so long as the teacher is clear about whether he or she is in 'didactic' or 'facilitator' mode. That is, if it is more appropriate for the group to work things out for themselves, it is time to switch to the 'say little, think hard' mode.

Honesty and openness remain important if trust is to develop. It is likely that teachers/facilitators will not know everything that they are asked or encounter, but they should not be afraid to admit it. Role-modelling how to find answers is an important aspect of the role.

Involve all members. What each member says should be carefully monitored. It is important that one or two people with forthright opinions should not dominate the group. Some quieter members think deeply and can contribute remarkably profound comments, if they have the opportunity. Alternatively, a quiet group member may be thinking of other things or be too shy to speak. There is an element of the 'ringmaster' role in being a small group facilitator, as sometimes groups need help to allow all members to have equal rights and roles. There is an art to doing this, as it is important not to discourage the loud ones too much. Instead the facilitator should rotate chairmanship of the group, intervene to ask quieter members for their views, and encourage groups to allocate tasks and air time equally.

Seek feedback. The facilitator should seek feedback from the group on his/her own performance as facilitator. It is important to establish a feeling of 'safety in receiving feedback' within the group. One way of fostering this is for the facilitator to be self-critical, when appropriate, and to ask for feedback from group members. As with the reverse, criticism should be constructive and able to be acted on.

Assessment in small groups

While the general rules of assessment are similar, there are a couple of important variations. Group members are often able to make sound assessments of the progress of each other, even if it is usually by comparison with that of their own progress. The trick is to use this feature constructively to help individual group members to learn. The key to success lies in the development of appropriate group dynamics and in ensuring that feedback from group members is given appropriately.

When group members work well together and trust each other's judgements, they will accept constructive criticism more readily. However, the rules of feedback should still be followed, with the minor modifications listed in Box 9.3. The only person allowed to make negative comments is the individual commenting on his or her own performance. All other group members should make positive and encouraging comments (e.g. 'I really like the way you said that'). Often individuals are rather negative about their own performance (self-confrontation theory, *see* Chapter 6) and feel much better when their peers confess that they have similar problems or underconfidence. The role of the facilitator is to monitor the feedback. This might necessitate intervention, either to reinforce what is being said or to raise concerns that have not been brought up by group members.

The best way to do this is through careful questioning, so that the concern is identified and must be addressed by the learners. For example, if the facilitator is concerned that, say, a prescription for a particular drug was not appropriate, the correct intervention is to say something like 'I see that you chose to prescribe [drug name] in this case. What benefits were you seeking?' This is usually enough to guide the individual learner and group members to this topic. The following discussion might cause the individual to consider a different drug or might satisfy your concerns that the correct drug was prescribed. Either way, the discussion would have been relevant and helpful to the learners.

Box 9.3 Group feedback skills

- Encourage comments, rather than criticisms
- The individual whose performance is being discussed comments first
- Other group members may make only positive or clarifying comments
- The group facilitator should raise concerns through skilled questioning
- Avoid leaving issues 'in the air'. Either address them now or arrange a later time

---

The most common role of group assessment is in formative assessment. However, there is a potential role in end-of-attachment assessments. Group members can often provide a valuable perspective on the whole attachment performance of both each group member and of the group as a whole. The most valuable information gained will be about the group process, and details about which objectives were achieved or not yet achieved, rather than pass/fail decisions. The facilitator could also give the group a score for group function or performance.

Example 1: practice-based small groups of medical students

Medical schools now more frequently place students in community settings to practise and develop clinical and communication skills. The basics might be taught with manikins, models and simulated patients within the medical school, but the opportunities for practice with real patients are now better in general practice than in hospitals. This kind of attachment is different to the traditional general practice attachment because the students are more junior and they often attend in at least pairs, so that they learn from each other.

The most common model for this in Australia is for students, either singly or in pairs, to attend general practices regularly to interview patients and practise clinical examination skills under the supervision of a GP tutor. Medical schools in London (Murray *et al.*, 1997) have adopted an interesting small group version of this. Students as early as second year are attached for a term of several weeks to an approved group practice in the suburbs. This requires attendance for half a day per week at the same time. One of the GPs has no personal clinical case-load for the half-day, devoting all his or her time to the students. The session commences with a short meeting, during which learning objectives for the session are reviewed. The session topic is known well in advance, so that all are prepared.

For this example, the topic is neurological examination skills. The students would have participated in a hospital-based tutorial on this, guided by a neurology registrar. Following the initial meeting, the students practise the examination skills on each other, receiving feedback from each other and from the GP tutor. When the tutor is satisfied, the students are allocated in pairs to some regular practice patients with known abnormal neurological signs. They take a history from and examine a patient, then reform into the larger group to present their patient in some detail to their tutor and colleagues. The discussion focuses on symptoms and signs, but also covers a range of other clinical issues such as diagnosis and management. Teaching quality assurance is conducted by the attendance once per term of a member of the academic general practice department to observe a tutorial.

Because the same group attends the same general practice for several weeks, group members and the tutor get to know each other quite well. Students recognise that general practice is the repository of a lot of interesting patients and problems, and GP tutors feel like part of the teaching team. This model could also operate in Australia, so long as GP tutors were paid sufficiently, as they are in London.

Example 2: practice-based small groups in vocational training

Practice-based small groups in vocational training are a little different because attachments are long term and almost always one learner to a single practice. However, there are usually several peers at the same stage in larger communities, so it should be possible to bring learners together at regular intervals for interactive sessions. This is of course the basis of GP registrar group meetings that are common in most vocational training schemes.

However, the usual format is for GP registrars to attend a central facility, often a hospital meeting room or training programme office, to discuss clinical cases. Variations on this theme provide much more interesting learning opportunities. These include:

- Move the registrar's meeting to one of the teaching practices, so that a small group meets within a practice. Using a different practice each time potentially increases the diversity of patients and approaches encountered. The GP registrar from that practice presents one or more patients for discussion. Ideally, the presentations reflect learning points that might be based on interesting or challenging cases. Each patient could be interviewed or examined by other group members, if that would bring out interesting symptoms or signs. The host GP supervisor would monitor the group process.

- A group critical incident analysis (*see* Chapter 8). The best format for this is for each learner to present a critical incident case, such that all will respect the feelings of the others and be supportive. Registrars are often pleasantly surprised at the relief they find in the resulting mutual support.

- Take the group to a different community setting: there are many different community healthcare settings, all of which could enrich learning. One example is to take the group to a nursing home, where each GP registrar interviews/examines a patient and then presents them to the larger group. Careful prior selection of cases ensures that a desired range of clinical topics is covered. Remember to obtain permission from staff and relatives.

- Take the group on an experiential outing. This is a more adventurous version of the previous category. Wandering around a supermarket with a nutritionist looking at the content and prices of common foodstuffs is a powerful method of learning about the affordability and nutritional value of family meals, recommended diets and dietary fads. Attending an optician for optical tests is an eye-opening experience for those who have not done this before. Similarly, visiting a physiotherapy practice for some mobilisation or ultrasound provides an opportunity to see common treatments from the perspective of patients. A GP should always participate in these sessions to ensure the relevance to actual practice. Further examples of community visits are listed in Table 9.1.

- Encourage registrars to form a 'peer review group'. This involves a relatively stable group of registrars meeting regularly for a period of time to discuss issues in common. The model is based on one which has been found to be particularly relevant for experienced GPs who want to monitor standards and quality of practice, and has been used widely to develop or adapt clinical practice guidelines (Grol and Lawrence, 1995). Issues more relevant to registrars might be working on similar practice projects (*see* Chapter 10) or preparation for examinations. An added advantage of encouraging this method with registrars is that it will familiarise participants with a method that they are likely to encounter later in their careers.

The key ingredients here are learner control and experience. Such sessions are a useful adjunct to other teaching and learning strategies. There is, of course, no reason why these 'fun' outings could not be used with medical students, depending on their learning objectives and level of learning.

Table 9.1 Examples of community-based experiences for learners. All should be facilitated by a GP

Location	Resource person	Objectives
Supermarket	Nutritionist	Cost of nutritious foods Food fads Product labelling Food additives
Optometrist practice	Optometrist	Services provided Experiencing testing
Physiotherapy practice	Physiotherapist	Services provided Experiencing therapy
Pathology laboratory	Pathologist, technicians	Cost of common tests Most relevant tests Accessing advice
Pharmacy	Pharmacist	Costs of drugs What advice they give Monitoring poly-pharmacy
Funeral parlour	Funeral director	Services provided Cost of dying Dying at home Cremation certificates

Distance sometimes impedes the capacity for a group of an appropriate size to meet. This can be overcome in regional and rural programmes by the use of multi-point video conferences that join up to eight to ten GP registrars in four or five sites for case presentations. Facilitation skills are a little different in this medium, because not all participants are visible on screen at the same time. Depending on the system, voice from a site switches the screen of all participants to the camera at that site, so those who talk most dominate the screen. This can make learning more passive for those at other sites. Hence it is important to monitor participation and ensure that all have an opportunity to contribute (Sen Gupta *et al.*, 1998).

Summary

This chapter has provided a brief overview of how to facilitate small group learning. This skill will be required more often in practice-based teaching as institutions move more of their educational activities to community-based healthcare facilities. Small group dynamics in learning situations are not dissimilar to those in other small groups, so skills acquired from this section should be applicable in other group settings.

Further reading

Grol R and Lawrence M (1995) *Quality Improvement by Peer Review*. Oxford General Practice Series 32. Oxford: Oxford University Press.
   While not directly relevant to GP registrar learning, the methods and principles presented in the book are a useful guide for those willing to encourage the concept with their group of registrars.

Whitman N (1990) *Creative Medical Teaching*. Salt Lake City, Utah: Department of Family and Preventive Medicine, University of Utah School of Medicine.
Crammed with innovative ideas about how to start and maintain group dynamics, this is a book to be dipped into from time to time rather than read from cover to cover. Topics are listed from A–Z and are extensively cross-referenced.

Chapter 10

Projects and audits

Knowledge advances by steps, not leaps.

Thomas Babington Macaulay, 1828

More than just clinical skills

Training for general practice is more than just training for a clinical role. Increasingly, other demands are placed on general practitioners. For example, we are expected to participate in some form of practice analysis as part of continuing education and quality assurance. We are also asked often by other organisations to participate in practice-based research projects. Some find these tasks onerous, as few have been trained to perform them well. If these issues are part of current general practice, then they should be included in training for general practice, particularly at the more advanced levels.

Projects and audits should not be conducted without a clear and desirable purpose. Both are powerful forms of inquiry, but they are time-consuming. For most GPs, such inquiry should be focused on issues of clinical care that are relevant to the practice. In particular, computerised information management systems make audits easy to conduct, but if the response to results is 'who cares?', it should not have been done.

Learners should be encouraged to engage in some form of inquiry during longer and more advanced attachments. The benefits are that, in addition to learning something of clinical relevance, they will learn some generic inquiry skills that will be useful later. Further, finding answers to questions (a simple definition of research?) that are relevant to clinical practice makes general practice much more interesting and satisfying. This chapter should help both learner and supervisor gain the most benefit from a practice-based clinical project.

Supervising learners' projects

Supervisors do not need a research degree to assist a learner to achieve a satisfying result, but it helps if they have personally conducted some form of inquiry. One of the nice features of learner projects is that they can be conducted with flexibility of timing and location. The steps to follow are simple: select a topic, find out what is already known about the topic, select the most appropriate methods, analyse and interpret the results, and report the results.

What topic?

The first step is for the learner to identify an issue worth exploring. The issue should be of interest to the learner and preferably of clinical relevance to the practice. Often the hardest part is the beginning, because the right question is the key to what follows.

Almost any aspect of clinical practice could be the subject of a project or audit, but it is best to find one that is relevant to your practice. A tip is to think about an issue which the textbooks say is correct, but which is more difficult to achieve in the real world of general practice. Above all, supervisors should try to have topics selected that they know they would like answered. A list of topics commonly chosen by GP registrars is given in Box 10.1.

Box 10.1 Common topics chosen for practice audits by learners

- Immunisation rates of practice patients
- Rates of eligible women with a Pap smear during the last two years
- Markers of diabetes care (e.g. HbA1c)
- Drugs prescribed for hypertension
- Investigations ordered
- Nature of referral pattern

What is already known about this issue?

Sometimes good ideas have been thought of before and researched satisfactorily. It helps to see what other projects have explored. Training programme offices often keep lists of registrar projects and, of course, Medline and other databases should be searched. Even if others have explored the issue, it might be interesting to see if the answer is the same in the supervisor's practice. On the other hand, if the results are already known, another topic might be more interesting and useful.

What methods should be used?

The search of other projects and the literature should have given some idea of the appropriate methods. What is wanted is a way of collecting information that helps answer the question; the simpler, the better. A common and achievable method is some form of audit of clinical cases. For example, information could be extracted from patient records (a lot of work!) or collected prospectively from the next, say 50, clinical encounters of a relevant kind. The number chosen might be important, so if it is planned to use statistics, advice may need to be sought. The nearest academic department of general practice should be able to assist. A useful book that is often recommended to university student researchers is that by Howard and Sharp (1994).

Interpretation and conclusion: the 'so what' factor

The results should answer the original question and produce a meaningful result. If so, congratulations! If not, learners should not worry. Rather they should be encouraged to think about possible reasons for the indecisive results. It may be that the methods were inappropriate, the number studied too small, or that real life does not imitate *in vitro* research. Quite often projects raise new or more precise issues that should be addressed in the future, and so still contribute to knowledge and understanding. If nothing else, the learner will have gained some experience in conducting projects.

Reporting

Regardless of the results, it is important to let others know about the project. Newsletters and meetings of the practice or the training programme are appropriate avenues. More formal publication may be appropriate, depending on the results.

Examples of practice-based projects

Two examples of practice-based projects are provided to guide supervisors and learners. The examples are fictitious, but illustrate that a project can lead the learner on an interesting journey, which will provide experience in thinking about and managing a project as well as provide a clinically relevant result. The results would not necessarily be true for all practices, and the projects are too small to provide answers to some very important questions about immunisation or diabetes management, but that was not their purpose. Both would help learners to understand principles of immunisation programmes or diabetes management much better and would succeed in focusing the attention of practice staff on how they manage common and important clinical conditions. Should they decide to make changes to routines, the studies could be repeated in a few months to see if anything had changed. This kind of study, involving any common or important clinical condition, is worth conducting in any general practice.

Example 1: Practice performance in tetanus booster vaccination

This project might be suitable for a medical student or relatively junior GP registrar in a short-term attachment of about one month. This topic was chosen because:

- vaccination programmes are an important strategy in illness prevention
- recent publicity indicates that fewer adults have current tetanus immunity than is desired.

Methods

All patients over the age of 18 presenting to the practice over two weeks will be asked at the reception desk to complete a small questionnaire prior to seeing all practice doctors. The questionnaire seeks information on last date of tetanus vaccination, their understanding of their current immune status (immune, not immune, uncertain). They will hand completed questionnaires to the doctor and will be offered immunisation if immune status is uncertain or poor. (Please note that practices with computerised records could extract this information on the entire practice population more easily.)

Results

Of 410 patients (58% of the practice population) presenting during the two-week period, 373 (91%) consented and handed in a completed questionnaire. A total of

221 (59%) respondents believed that they had had a tetanus booster within the previous five years, with percentages ranging from 88% in the 18–24 age group to 44% in the over-65 age group. This compares with an estimate of 43% having current immunity to tetanus in the whole community. Immune status was documented in only 78% (of the 59% of those who believed they had had a tetanus booster) of patient records. Overall, 131 (35%) of respondents were uncertain of their immune status.

Conclusions

A higher proportion of the practice population appears to have current tetanus immunity than the broader community. However, the proportion is still low. Practice procedures should be amended to offer the vaccine to more patients and to document this better.

Recommendations

1 The practice should develop and implement a programme to encourage more patients to have a tetanus booster.
2 Practice staff should be reminded to improve documentation of immune status of patients.

Example 2: Diabetes management in this general practice

This project might be suitable for a more advanced GP registrar, who is in an attachment of several months. The project aims to explore the management of patients with diabetes in this practice in order to determine if acceptable care is provided. This topic was chosen because:

- diabetes causes substantial morbidity and cost to both people and the community
- it is common in general practice
- the registrar sees several patients with long-standing diabetes who do not seem to be doing well. Is the practice doing all that it could do?
- practice members support the idea and will help.

What is already known?

A great deal, but much of it seems to refer to 'ideal' management in specialised units. Plenty of protocols are available, but there is little information on clinical outcomes.

Methods

A retrospective and prospective study of all diabetics seen in the practice during the next three months will be conducted. This is estimated to be about 20 patients. All practice doctors will complete a data sheet as they see each diabetic patient. The data sheet will collate data such as:

- date of encounter, number of consultations in last 12 months
- seen by endocrinologist?
- age, gender, type of diabetes, duration of diabetes
- number and type of current health problems
- weight, blood pressure, peripheral circulation, vision

- urinalysis, blood sugar level on the day, HbA1c, renal function
- drugs being prescribed and taken
- dates of last contact with dietitian, ophthalmologist, podiatrist
- estimate by GP of the motivation and degree of compliance of each patient.

These data will be used to compile a detailed description of how this practice manages diabetes and to see if the care matches available protocols.

Results

The practice has the expected number of diabetic patients, as predicted by population figures. Most non-insulin-dependent diabetes mellitus (NIDDM) patients are overweight (mean body mass index >30). Most are normotensive (50% are on medication), about 5% have signs of peripheral vascular disease. Only about 50% have seen dietitians, ophthalmologists and podiatrists during the last 12 months. About 30% have high HbA1c levels, most of whom were regarded by the GPs as having poor compliance with management.

Conclusions

In general, the care of diabetic patients conforms to accepted guidelines. Not all relevant information is documented in practice records. More use could be made of other health professionals. There seems to be a core of NIDDM patients who are difficult to motivate.

Recommendations

1 To improve documentation of important indicators of diabetes care.
2 To increase the proportion of patients seen by an ophthalmologist within 12 months to 90%.
3 To obtain outside advice about how to motivate non-compliant patients.

Summary

This chapter describes how learners can participate in projects and audits in order to gain both project skills and relevant clinical knowledge. Topics should be of interest to the learner and of clinical or professional relevance to their practice. The future of general practice requires that clinicians participate in defining and improving quality of care.

Further reading

Hays RB, Bushfield M and Strasser R (1993) Encouraging trainee general practitioners to conduct research. *Postgraduate Education for General Practice.* 4 (2): 117–20.
   A guide to giving learners the enthusiasm and the skills to commence small projects.
Howard K and Sharp JA (1989) *The Management of a Student Research Project.* Aldershot: Gower Publishing.
   A popular textbook with university research students that has been revised many times since it was first published in 1983. It provides detailed advice about how to achieve methodological rigour. Probably more detailed than most medical students and GP registrars would require for small projects, but worthwhile reading for supervisors with an interest in practice-based projects.

Howie JGR (1989) *Research in General Practice* (2e). London: Chapman and Hall.
    One of the most experienced GP researchers explains how general practitioners can contribute more effectively to the pursuit of answers to practical primary care questions.
Pringle M, Bradley CP, Carmichael CM, Wallis H and Moore A (1995) *Significant Event Auditing.* RCGP Occasional Paper 50. London: Royal College of General Practitioners.
    More or less the definitive guide to how to achieve high-quality audits in the UK context. This is available at www.rcgp.org.uk.

Chapter 11

Documenting learning achievement

> We learn so little and forget so much.
>
> Sir John Davies, 1599

An overview of clinical teaching

A theme of this manual is that there is no single method of passing on knowledge and skills to learners. Instead, a skilled clinical supervisor takes an eclectic approach, using strategies that suit the needs of the learner, the skills of the supervisor and the strengths of the particular strategy. If this approach is adopted, then learners will have quite varied learning experiences. There will be variations in topic content, as each learner enters each stage of learning with different prior experiences and levels of knowledge. There will be variations in the sequencing of topic content, depending on what learners encounter during their clinical attachments, and there will be variations in the extent to which particular teaching and learning strategies are used.

However, over the duration of an entire training course, learners are expected to reach a similar end-point and to have mastered a similar range of curriculum issues. It is difficult for educational organisations to document so many different pathways to the end-point, so it makes sense for learners to document their own pathway. There are two reasons for this form of documentation. The most important is that learners can monitor their own progress towards covering the entire curriculum. In an adult learning context, learners carry substantial responsibility for this. Through regular discussion with supervisors, gaps or weaknesses can be identified and remedial plans made. For this reason alone, learners should be encouraged to collect information relevant to their training. The second reason is for programme evaluation, or ensuring that the course has met its objectives. More on this issue is presented in Chapter 12.

This chapter presents information on how to assist learners to document learning achievement, which in turn helps supervisors understand their contribution to the professional development of others.

Learning portfolios

A topical name for the documentation by learners of their learning is a *learning portfolio*. Over the last five years learning portfolios have assumed a much more prominent role in medical education. Most medical students and registrars are now expected to maintain some form of learning portfolio, and many medical schools and professional bodies now even assess them summatively. Further, revalidation in the UK now requires all medical practitioners to keep some form of learning portfolio, although the precise use of the information had not been resolved at the time of writing.

Any discussion about learning portfolios soon becomes bogged down in definitions and descriptions of just what is meant by a learning portfolio. In concept, it is simply a folder into which learners place descriptions of what they have learned and any evidence of achievement of learning goals. Although initially thought to be primarily of value for the 'hard to measure' attributes, such as personal and professional behaviours, learning portfolios are increasingly being used to assess a wider range of learner attributes, from knowledge and skills to personal and professional development, becoming closer to a format for '360 degree' assessment of learners.

The contents vary widely, but might include:

- A curriculum outline, in terms of both content and process, against which progress can be checked. This should include learning objectives for knowledge, skills and attitudes, and lists of clinical conditions that should be encountered, clinical skills that should be mastered and procedural skills that should be observed or performed. Further, there should be an indication of what should be achieved at each stage (or module) of the course.
- Copies of learning plans negotiated with the supervisor.
- A record (log diary) of clinical cases encountered.
- A record of clinical skills performed satisfactorily.
- A record of practical procedures performed satisfactorily.
- A record of attendance at educational events, possibly including topics, venues, speakers and perceived value.
- A record of specific teaching and learning strategies employed during training. These might include sitting in, external clinical teaching visits, videotape review, patient record review, etc. Copies of formative assessments by supervisors would be helpful.
- A record of training adviser interviews with supervisors and mentors throughout training. These should provide evidence that learning has progressed by indicating topics that have been mastered and those that require further work.
- Copies of specific assessments are required by the educational institution, as with in-training assessment.
- Reflective comments on how the learner is managing the workload, encountering and mastering (or not) the curriculum, and achieving (or not) the learning objectives.

This documentation is labour-intensive, but is useful in ensuring that an appropriate range of common, important, chronic or complex problems is encountered. Periodic recording can reduce the perception of high workload as well as ensure that the recording is more accurate and any reflective comments are more relevant.

Depending on the preferences of individual learners, a learning portfolio has the potential to be large and perhaps cumbersome. This is most likely to happen when learners simply place everything in the portfolio without any consideration of what it means or how useful it may be in the future.

The reflective component is arguably the most controversial. Reflection may not come easily to some, and is probably a skill that develops as part of the capacity to be a more self-directed adult learner. Junior medical students often prefer a highly structured, 'fill in the numbers' model, whereas experienced professionals will tend to want to create their own structure and format. The nature of reflection also needs consideration. The issue to be reflected on is the progress towards achieving the learning objectives. This is not really a personal diary of life's experience (that may be useful but perhaps should be separate from what is submitted for review), but about identifying strengths and weaknesses and ways of filling in gaps.

In summary, a learning portfolio could contain just about anything of value to the learner. Over time it can develop into a personalised 'textbook' that encompasses the personal learning journey of the learner. This can be useful for revision prior to final examinations and even as a complement to a curriculum vitae or résumé in job applications. The responsibility for collecting and maintaining these pieces of information rests with the learner.

The format of learning portfolios

The traditional model is paper-based, but this is dating rapidly as 'e-learning' becomes more feasible. Most of the curriculum material of universities and professional bodies is now web-accessible, as are log diary and assessment forms. Some learners adopt newer technology rapidly and should be allowed to have electronic versions of the materials and maintain their learning portfolio on computers, including laptop and hand-held devices. A written component will be necessary unless signed assessment forms are scanned in as non-changeable documents, but having at least some of the material in electronic format can assist with both recording and portability. Novice learners may need a more explicitly defined structure and format until they become familiar with the concept. Therefore there will be a substantial difference between what junior medical students and advanced GP registrars have to include in their learning portfolios.

Purposes of the documentation

Learning portfolios can have more than one purpose, and the intended purpose influences the design and contents. The primary purpose of learning portfolios at the current time is to augment the assessment of learning progress of individual learners through placing together a wide range of pieces of information that can inform and help monitor learning progress. This is essentially a formative process that is managed primarily by individual learners, but is helped by regular discussion with supervisors and professional educators. Novice learners can be guided in how to use learning portfolios to become more self-directed, adult learners.

More recently learning portfolios have been assessed summatively, particularly for curriculum domains covering ethical, personal and professional development issues. However, they are now being used more widely as another source of evidence for achieving learning objectives related to knowledge and skills. This is discussed further in Chapter 3.

The third purpose of learning portfolios is to guide programme evaluation. Educational institutions might also want to collect information about learning progress to help determine if the curriculum is being covered. One interpretation of a finding that a high proportion of learners do not achieve particular experiences or levels of knowledge and skill is that either the learning experience or the assessment process is flawed.

As the summative assessment and programme evaluation roles are quite different tasks to that of guiding individual learners, questions of ownership and access may arise. The principles of in-training assessment (*see* Chapter 3) re-emerge here to guide the rights of learners and educational institutions. Learners should be free (and encouraged) to maintain their own learning portfolio, to which the institution should have access only with the permission of the learners. Documentation required by the institution for in-training assessment purposes should be defined clearly and only material explicitly collected for that purpose should be included in the documentation going to the institution. Material wanted for programme evaluation is much less controversial, as this should not be harmful to learners, but may still require separate collection. Hence, there may be need for a two-volume learning portfolio – one solely for the learner and one for the institution. This approach would require the approval of a human ethics committee.

Measurement of learning portfolios

To understand the role of learning portfolios in assessment requires a conceptual leap rather like that of understanding the role of objective structured clinical examinations (OSCEs). Just as an OSCE is a format, rather than an assessment method, so too are learning portfolios a format and not a method. One of the theoretical strengths of OSCEs and learning portfolios is that they include a range of assessments of different attributes by several different people, combining to produce a valid and reliable overall decision.

In practice, however, much more is known about how to achieve strong validity and reliability in OSCEs than with learning portfolios. The validity and reliability of the overall score will depend on those of the individual components being assessed. It is difficult to give a numerical score to personal and professional behaviours, so assessment relies on judgements. Assessors should be experienced educators trained in learning portfolio assessment methods.

The supervisor's role in documentation

Supervisors are with each learner for only a portion of his or her entire training course, and may feel that they are not in a position to make much of a contribution to such a long-term record. This, however, is not correct and represents a misunderstanding of the role of supervisors. The learner's journey involves contact with many supervisors in different settings, and all can contribute both to the learner's professional development and to constructing a learning portfolio that reflects that professional development during the entire course. Hence they should be aware of the expectations of the educational institution and ensure that they are able to meet the needs of both learner and institution. That is, care must be taken to help learners to collect as much information and documentation as they find helpful in their personal learning portfolios, while the documentation required for either in-training assessment or programme evaluation is collected for the institution. As a rule, much of the institutional information might be of value to learners (unless the institution requests that this not be done), whereas information for learners should not be passed on to institutions without the permission of learners.

GP supervisors are unlikely to be the decision makers about scores and progress – that is more likely to be done by academic staff within the university or training programme. However, GP supervisors are in a very good position to observe how the learners behave in professional settings than are the central academic staff who make the decisions. They should be able to see where the learners' strengths and weaknesses lie across all the curriculum domains, including knowledge, skills and attitudes. Whereas a learner might do well in an observed simulated patient encounter in a skills laboratory, a GP supervisor might observe poor knowledge, poor clinical reasoning, poor dress standards, poor attendance or even rudeness to patients.

Having identified any weaknesses or gaps, the primary role of the GP supervisor is to try to remediate any identified weaknesses. This conforms with the mostly formative role of learning portfolios. The more accurate the information and the more skilled the supervisor is at providing feedback and motivating change, the more effective will be the formative assessment.

However, if that fails, it is very important that GP supervisors document both the weaknesses and the failed remediation for the central academic staff, who are then responsible for further remediation and/or decisions about progress. The reporting should be limited to clear, non-judgemental descriptions of the troublesome issues or behaviours. It is then up to the central academic staff to make a judgement, generally based on feedback from more than one supervisor. Learners with problems almost always attract similar comments from all or most supervisors, providing course organisers with sufficient evidence to justify calling in the learner for counselling.

However, this system will work only where concerns are communicated. Many GP supervisors are reluctant to communicate concerns in case 'it is just me – we seem to have a personality clash'. If several supervisors fail to report similar concerns, the learner will probably continue with persistent problems. Neither the learner nor society is done any favour by silence.

Using the learning portfolio

While the supervisors are hosting learners in their practices, they also play an important role in helping learners to review their progress towards achievement of learning objectives. It might be worthwhile revisiting the material on the model of learning supervision in Chapter 4. The learning portfolio can facilitate clinical supervision, because it should make clear what has been achieved to date, and what topics and experiences are missing. This information guides negotiation of future learning goals. It may be possible to arrange for particular patients to be seen by the learner or for opportunities to practise particular clinical skills or perform particular practical procedures. Achievement of learning objectives during the current stay should be 'signed off' by supervisors, thus providing useful information for the next supervisor.

Summary

Learning portfolios are an evolving documentation of the progress and achievement of learners during a training course. They can have different structures, content and purposes. Increasingly, they are regarded as a valuable source of information to guide summative assessment. Supervisors should be clear about precisely what is required for their learners' learning portfolios, and understand their role in helping learners monitor progress. Supervisors should also be clear about the purposes of the documentation, to avoid a possible conflict of responsibilities towards learners and the educational institution.

Further reading

Royal College of General Practitioners (1993) *Portfolio-based Learning.* RCGP Occasional Paper 63. London: RCGP.
A more detailed description of the development and application of learning portfolios in postgraduate general practice education.
Snadden D, Thomas ML, Griffin EM and Hudson H (1996) Portfolio-based learning and general practice vocational training. *Medical Education.* **30** (2): 148–52.
Describes the practical use of learning portfolios in a concise manner.

Chapter 12

Evaluating teaching and learning

> Experience is the name everyone gives to their mistakes.
>
> Oscar Wilde, 1892

Introduction

This chapter presents a brief overview of approaches to seeking answers to the question: 'How well is this practice performing in its role as a teaching and learning practice?'

To do this the text returns to educational theory to demonstrate that evaluation is an essential part of teaching and learning. It also provides practical examples of how to conduct evaluation of teaching and learning. Much of the material might be more relevant to the staff of an educational organisation rather than to individual practice supervisors, but the principles should also be understood and adopted by those individuals, as they stand to gain the most from their professional development. Finally, common practical evaluation methods (and their difficulties and pitfalls) are presented to demonstrate their application to practice-based teaching.

Why evaluate?

It is difficult to stop learners learning, although more difficult to ensure that learners are proceeding down the right learning pathways. It is true that practice-based teaching and learning offer a variety of learning opportunities, with a variety of clinical problems that present in differing sequences. Further, general practice is such a diverse discipline that one would expect, even desire, different outcomes for different learners. Nevertheless, it is all too easy to assume correct points will be reached if each learner is simply allowed to follow their own individual and unique pathway, relying on the formative and summative assessment programmes to provide the necessary guiding information.

It is not that this view is invalid, but rather it is more relevant to the assessment of learning than teaching. Teaching is an active role, even if the model of supervision presented in this manual appears to be a less obvious role than in traditional didactic teaching. Indeed, clinical supervision is more difficult than giving a lecture, because it requires the skills of monitoring learning progress within a close relationship. There are many ways in which this process can be less than optimal. For this reason alone evaluation is essential.

In this book a broad definition of educational evaluation is adopted: the measurement of progress towards meeting agreed educational objectives. In the context of practice-based teaching there are two main reasons for measuring such progress. The first is that teachers need to receive feedback on their skills for their professional development as teachers. Teachers are also learners and through feedback they will become better teachers and better clinicians in their own professional development journeys. The second reason is for programme evaluation. Educational institutions have a responsibility to ensure that learners are receiving the best possible facilitation of learning and that the educational objectives of the programme have been achieved. Learners and funders of education have a right to expect value for the effort and expense. Institutional programme evaluation is usually a condition of funding for educational programmes.

Concepts and principles of educational evaluation

By definition, evaluation is *measurement against a standard, for a purpose*. However, this is a rather narrow definition, as it implies that there is always a precise standard against which to measure. In educational evaluation, the aim is usually to measure progress against stated educational objectives. Often there are no precise standards for this, so educational evaluation methods must accommodate this.

Evaluation of teaching and learning should adopt the following principles:

- Standards should be criterion-referenced (*see* Chapter 3), where available. Standards should reflect an agreed understanding of what is required, rather than being better or worse than what others do.
- The focus should be on quality improvement. The purpose of the evaluation is to achieve continuous improvement of teaching and learning. The philosophy should be that all teaching and all teachers can improve, similar to that which underpins clinical quality assurance programmes.
- Evaluation should be built into the design of the teaching programme. Evaluation of teaching should not be regarded as an afterthought, but as an integral part of the entire teaching and learning programme. Prospective evaluation is preferable to retrospective evaluation, as information collection is easier and the results are more powerful.
- Information collection should be efficient. Where possible, the evaluation framework should use information gathered for other purposes, so that teachers and learners are not bothered by too frequent requests for information, some of it not essential to the clinical supervision model. However, additional information may still need to be sought to address specific evaluation questions.

Evaluation hierarchies

Evaluation is a generic term, which can be applied to different issues in different contexts (i.e. not simply educational contexts). It can also produce results that show variation in the degree to which objectives are achieved. A common general model of the evaluation of quality of healthcare, proposed by Donabedian (1988), includes *structure, process* and *outcome* measures. (As true outcomes are difficult to define and measure, an intermediate step is to measure *impacts*, or short-term results that contribute to outcomes. This is also a useful concept in educational evaluation.) Structural evaluation provides information about what could happen, whereas outcome evaluation provides information about what has happened; hence this model could be viewed as an education evaluation hierarchy.

Structural evaluation

Structural evaluation is performed by focusing on *what* is done. If teachers and learners have adopted the procedures suggested in this manual, then structural evaluation is simple. Structural issues include the recruitment of teaching practices and teachers, curriculum and assessment procedures, and any documentation relevant to how the teaching programme is established. Some of these structural issues are listed in Box 12.1.

The level of evaluation here is low, in that these structural aspects might be either present or absent. Most could be assessed qualitatively, as the quality might vary from poor to excellent. Detailed analyses are logistically difficult and are probably not appropriate for routine use, although periodic assessment of the quality of teaching plans and learning portfolios is a good idea. However, the presence of high-quality structural documentation does not necessarily mean that a programme will be delivered well or will achieve desired outcomes.

Box 12.1 Measurable structural evaluation issues

1 A clear curriculum, with learning objectives, a blueprint and identified teaching and learning strategies. This should be readily available to teachers and learners.
2 A clear and open assessment programme, so that all participants know what will be assessed (i.e. domains and components of competence), how this will be assessed (format) and when it will be assessed. Formative and summative assessment should be clearly identified, particularly where there is in-training assessment.
3 A sufficient number of teaching practices that offer appropriate clinical and educational opportunities for learners. This might include the presence of educational resources such as facilities for learners to see patients, a small library and a computer with internet access. Ideally, each practice should maintain a current teaching plan.
4 A sufficient number of trained practice-based teachers and a continuing programme of teacher training.
5 Learners maintain a current and comprehensive learning portfolio that describes in detail their individual learning journey.

Process evaluation

This focuses on *how* things are done. It might include how often and how well particular learning strategies are used. Teaching plans and learning portfolios play a role here, as they are evolving documents that should describe progress towards achieving learning objectives. Teachers might be observed in their practice-based teaching roles by academic staff. Box 12.2 lists a range of relevant process issues. Detailed analyses are resource-intensive, but should be conducted periodically. The level of evaluation is higher than for structural evaluation, as good implementation should lead to better outcomes, but it is still descriptive and does not guarantee good outcomes.

Box 12.2 Process issues that are potentially useful in evaluation

1 Learning pathways of individual learners, e.g. the number and sequence of particular experiences.
2 Practice teaching plans. These should reflect continuing development and improvement of practice-based teaching.
3 Learning portfolios. These should reflect a continuing learning process, particularly from the perspective of the learner. Learners would need to consent to the use of their learning portfolios for evaluation purposes.
4 Formative assessment. Both learners and institutions should document progress towards meeting objectives. There should be regular identification of learning objectives and evidence of remediation. There is overlap with the analysis of learning portfolios.
5 Self-assessment, peer assessment and tutor assessment. Perceptions by learners and teachers on aspects such as enjoyment, value, coverage of curriculum, etc.

Impact and outcome evaluation

This focuses on evidence that learners are progressing towards achievement of learning objectives and a good outcome. Impact and outcome measures are usually 'harder' than structural and process measures, in that they should be measures of achievement of particular components of competence that contribute to overall competence, even if they alone do not indicate this. Examples include scores on a range of assessment instruments that are used for formative and in-training assessment.

Outcome evaluation focuses on measuring achievement of the intended result of the education programme. This often means an attempt to evaluate the whole package, or at least a number of different aspects of the whole package. Results of summative assessment (the end-point of training) might appear to be the most appropriate outcome assessment, as it is usually the accepted measure of achievement of competence of learners. However, summative assessment is somewhere between an impact and an outcome measure, because it rarely assesses performance of graduates in the real world after completion of training. The less congruence there is between curriculum design implementation and assessment, the further summative assessment results are from outcome evaluation.

Hence true outcome evaluation requires a much broader approach than is provided by relying on summative assessment results. Some in-training assessment procedures that measure workplace performance (e.g. videotaped consultations in advanced training, review of patient records, etc.) may reflect true performance better than usual competency assessment. True outcome measurement – measuring performance in the real world after graduation – is possible, but requires resource-intensive educational research. Hence this is attempted infrequently. Table 12.1 indicates the overlap between impact and outcome evaluation measures.

Table 12.1 Impact and outcome evaluation measures

Measure	Impact	Outcome
Performance of supervisors	++	−
Some formative assessment of learners	++	−
Some in-training assessment of learners	++	+
End-point summative assessment of learners	+	++
Performance after graduation of learners	+	+++

A hierarchy for educational evaluation methods

Another model hierarchy of evaluation specifically for medical educational evaluation is presented in Table 12.2. This proposes eight levels of evaluation (from nil to health outcomes-based) commonly seen in teaching evaluation. However, evaluations of teaching infrequently pass level five – the measurement of change in attitudes. This is partly because it is difficult to measure level 6 – change in behaviour – without adopting assessment of performance in actual practice, and even more difficult to measure level 7 – change in healthcare outcomes – because healthcare is complex. In principle, however, evaluations should attempt to measure change in behaviour and healthcare outcomes. There are some useful concepts here for evaluating education programmes at all levels.

Table 12.2 A hierarchy of evaluation of teaching (after Pitts *et al.*, 1995)

Level	Description of measures
0	Nil
1	Satisfaction
2	Educational objectives listed and coverage
3	Wider educational needs sought and coverage
4	Learning outcome assessed – knowledge or skills
5	Learning outcome assessed – attitudes change
6	Learning outcome assessed – change in behaviour
7	Health benefit outcomes – improvement in patient care

Evaluation of practice-based teaching

The remainder of this chapter focuses on the evaluation of practice-based teaching, because that is the likely interest of clinical supervisors. Supervisors might want to evaluate the teaching and learning in their own practices, either for personal interest and professional development, or to assist course organisers with more formal programme evaluation. Further reading is suggested for those who wish to exceed this scope.

A sound approach to evaluation is summarised in Box 12.3. The first step is to decide what is to be evaluated. The objectives of the practice attachment should act as a guide. There might be learning objectives, as previously discussed, and also teaching objectives, which would relate more to the roles and expectations of the supervisor than the learner. Some possible evaluation topics are listed in Box 12.4; note that these should be related to a specific level of learner and a specific context. For example, a learning objective relating to learners improving their communication skills through experience and feedback might translate into a teaching objective relating to helping learners improve communication skills through the provision of feedback using direct observation and videotape review.

Box 12.3 An approach to evaluation of practice-based teaching

Step 1   Select the aspect of practice-based teaching to be evaluated.
Step 2   Select the most appropriate measure.
Step 3   Select the most appropriate evaluation method.
Step 4   Link results to learning objectives and teaching objectives.

The second step is to select the most appropriate measure. This requires consideration of what would provide evidence that the objectives had been achieved. Continuing with the example of communication skills teaching, one could look for evidence that the teaching took place (structure), that the teaching was regarded as enjoyable, valued and effective (process), and that the learner actually progressed (impact/outcome). Progress could be measured by a communication skills rating scale. Serial measures (by both self and supervisor) should demonstrate improvement. Information about the performance of others at the same stage of training might be available for comparison.

The third step is to select an appropriate method. In the example of communication skills, this might be a review of videotaped consultations. Learners could also provide information about the perceived value of the learning methods and other aspects, such as technical and logistic aspects; this depends on what is decided in step one.

The final step is the interpretation of the results, which have most meaning when used to specifically address the objectives of the attachment and what is decided in step one. It is important not to try to use results to answer questions that were not addressed correctly. An example of inappropriate interpretation, staying with the example of communication skills, is claiming that videotape review is more or less effective than other forms of communication skills teaching. Individual learners and teachers might think that this is true, but comparative data from multiple teaching methods would be needed to address that issue.

Box 12.4 Some evaluation topics relevant to practice-based teaching

- Gaining understanding of the nature of general or rural practice
- Prescribing skills
- Communication skills
- Physical examination skills
- Practical procedural skills
- Practice management skills
- Information management skills

Some common evaluation methods

This section relates to step three in Box 12.3 and assumes that the topic and the most appropriate measure have been selected. Common evaluation methods include content analysis of existing documentation, administration of questionnaires and conducting interviews. These are discussed in more detail below.

Analysis of existing information

It is likely that most evaluation questions could be answered through analysis of the material already collected by practices, learners and course organisers. This may be recorded in a variety of instruments that record quantitative information, qualitative information, or both. Just what is done with the information depends on the specific issue being evaluated and the nature of the information collected.

At the level of structural evaluation, the question is the presence or absence of evidence that an appropriate teaching and learning environment existed. Teaching plans, teaching facilities, timetables, etc. provide the evidence about which a judgement is made. For process evaluation, the question relates to how well this teaching and learning environment functioned. The frequency of particular educational strategies, the number of patients seen and practical procedures performed, how well course content was covered, etc. provide evidence for this. For impact evaluation, the question is what resulted from the teaching and learning environment. The results of formative and in-training assessments are relevant here, particularly if there are serial assessments that demonstrate change: self-assessments, peer assessments, patient assessments and supervisor assessments. The analysis of serial assessments can provide both numerical evidence of change (if there are numerical scales) or descriptions of performance and change. True outcome evaluation is not easily addressed at the level of practice-based teaching.

Questionnaires

An evaluation question might require information that is not available from existing sources. One method of collecting additional information is to ask learners to complete a questionnaire. This would be of value if the questions concern aspects of the supervisor's teaching practice environment over a period of time, and involve several learners. In a sense, a questionnaire could be used to 'add together' perceptions of a series of learners or a series of patients. However, with small numbers of respondents, the ability to de-identify respondents is severely restricted, such that anonymity is difficult to attain. Hence, interpretation should be cautious.

Questionnaires are commonly used and often misused. A questionnaire is a highly structured method of gathering information. It has the advantage that it is easily administered, but the disadvantage that written words can be interpreted differently and clarification is not possible. These are potentially valuable sources of information, but are often poorly designed and interpreted. A poor questionnaire provides information that is either useless or irrelevant to the specific question in mind. Questionnaire design is a skill that few part-time evaluators will possess. Principles of questionnaire design include:

- careful selection of issues to be addressed. Avoid the temptation to ask more questions than are necessary
- precise and concise wording to avoid ambiguity
- careful layout to improve readability. Crowded questionnaires are more difficult to complete
- a balance between types of questions. For example, ticking response boxes is easy for respondents, but provides less information. Free responses provide more information, but are more difficult to complete
- piloting. All questionnaires should be completed by a small trial group of people to ensure that they are clear and unambiguous
- sampling. Ideally, questionnaires should be sent either to a whole population of respondents (where numbers are small) or to a random sample of respondents. The former is the usual method for small numbers of learners.

Interpreting questionnaire-generated information also provides some traps for the unwary. Questionnaires produce opinions and perceptions of respondents; these are not necessarily correct, or even factual. The larger the number of completed questionnaires, the more likely the results are to be applicable to a broader group. Also, questionnaires completed by learners in one practice will not necessarily reflect what is happening in another practice. However, questionnaires might provide information about the teaching and learning environment in a particular practice that is useful to the clinical supervisors in that practice. Those intending to use a questionnaire should seek advice from more experienced researchers.

Interviews

Interviewing learners, staff and patients about the teaching and learning environment can provide some rich information about a practice. An interviewer has the opportunity to respond to cues and explore these further. When conducted correctly, this method has the potential to provide the most valuable information about a teaching practice.

Interviews may be unstructured, semi-structured or tightly structured. The former is the most difficult, but potentially most valuable, while the latter is easier but may not provide much more information than a questionnaire. Interviews may also be of individuals, groups of similar individuals or groups of different categories of individuals. One of the best known forms of interview is a focus group.

However, the traps are deeper here than for questionnaires. Designing an interview pro forma is as difficult as designing questions for a questionnaire. Interviewing requires skills in small group dynamics and an ability to monitor progress towards group objectives. The interpretation of information from interviews requires qualitative analysis skills. These are skills that few general practitioners possess. The clinical supervisor should probably not be the interviewer or the interpreter, as he or she is one of the most important components of the teaching and learning environment and may find dispassionate objectivity difficult to achieve. Those interested in using interview methods should seek advice.

Evaluation in practice: an example

Box 12.5 presents a brief outline of a possible evaluation question and the information that might exist, or be collected additionally, to answer the question. The question is really three questions, as it addressed the meeting of the expectations of three different groups. It would be simpler to address only one of these questions, but all three are included just to exemplify the different information that might be collected. Much of the necessary information is listed as 'existing', but this would be true for some information only if teaching plans and learning portfolios existed and were maintained; this should indicate just how valuable such documents are in the evaluation of teaching and learning.

The method of analysis of information collected will depend on the nature of the information. Much of it will be purely descriptive, in that certain things did or did not happen. Where numerical data are available, these may be described with simple statistical methods, such as frequency counts and some description of mid-range values. Numbers of cases seen and learning activities experienced indicate the level of learning activity. Responses to Likert rating scales (*see* Chapter 3) might show a mean score of 3.3 on a 1–5 scale, and serial measures might show change in scores over time. Please note that mid-range values may be expressed as means, medians or modes; each has a particular meaning and application. For a more detailed explanation of how measurement theory affects rating scales, see Streiner and Norman (1993) or Foulkes *et al.* (1994). Qualitative information requires a more inductive analysis, with the aim of developing an understanding of how and why (or why not) teaching and learning occur in the practice. The views of different participants (learners, staff and patients) are valuable as they represent differing perspectives and might highlight information that is not obvious. In particular, agreement of differing perspectives (*triangulation*) usually means that the issue is significant.

Box 12.5 Example evaluation of a teaching practice

Evaluation question: How well does the learning experience meet the expectations of (Q1) the educational instution, (Q2) the learners and (Q3) the practice staff?

Methods: Comparison of structure, process and impact issues from the practice with the expectations of the educational institution. Measures are dictated by learning objectives of the attachment (e.g. understanding of general practice, consulting skills, confidence ratings, practical procedures, etc.)

Existing information
- Learning objectives of the practice attachment (from the educational institution)
- Practice teaching plan
- Learning portfolio (patients seen; skills and procedures performed; formative assessments from sitting in and video review; clinical topic tutorials, etc.)

Additional information (Q = question)
- Assessment of practice by academic staff from the educational institution (Q1)
- Assessment of practice by clinical supervisors from other teaching practices (Q1, 2 and 3)
- Assessment of practice by a panel of learners who have not worked in the practice (Q2)
- Interviews with learners (all for 1–2 years?) and practice staff (Q2 and 3)

Moving to the level of impact or outcome evaluation is more difficult. There are unlikely to be firm measures of what learners should have achieved at the completion of a practice attachment. Reflecting on the adult learning approach, learners will commence and complete practice attachments at different levels of achievement, although by the end of the whole course they should have mastered at least a core set of curriculum objectives. With this short-term approach to evaluation, impacts for the whole course are often regarded as outcomes of components of the course. Hence mastery of (say) prescribing skills – a component of competence assessed at the end of a training course – could be regarded as an outcome of a practice attachment early in vocational training. Potential outcome measures should be made obvious by the learning objectives of the attachment.

Summary

As was stated at the beginning, this chapter presents a brief overview of approaches to seeking answers to the question: 'How well is this practice performing in its role as a teaching and learning practice?' This is an important question and clinical supervisors should ask it of themselves often. A regular cycle of teaching and learning evaluation will develop teaching practices into 'learning organisations' that offer high-quality educational opportunities for learners and satisfying professional development for supervisors. After working through this chapter, readers will not be experts in evaluation methodology, but should understand the principles of educational evaluation and be able to apply them in their practice.

Further reading

Best JW and Kahn JV (1989) *Research in Education* (5e). Englewood Cliffs, NJ: Prentice-Hall.
    An overview of approaches to educational research and evaluation. Full of practical examples from classroom settings.

Donabedian A (1988) The quality of care: how can it be assessed? *Journal of the American Medical Association.* **260**: 1743–8.
    A clear explanation of the most often cited model of evaluation in healthcare.

Pitts J, Percy D and Coles C (1995) Evaluating teaching. *Education for General Practice.* **6**: 13–18.
    Describes a simple and meaningful hierarchy of evaluation in medical education.

Wadsworth Y (1992) *Do It Yourself Social Research.* Melbourne: Victorian Council of Social Service.
    Brief and practical advice on how to conduct qualitative research. It is easily understood by relatively novice researchers, but provides a sound approach.

A guide to the galaxy of education jargon

This chapter provides explanations of terms commonly used in educational and assessment circles. These are listed in alphabetical order, although some similar concepts are grouped.

Assessment is the measurement of particular attributes at a particular point in time.

    Formative assessment is assessment designed to inform learners about their progress towards achieving mastery of the course. In the context of the RACGP training programme, this means **feedback** and should be regarded as an integral part of teaching and learning. It includes observing, reviewing and informing learners about their progress towards mastering knowledge and skills.

    In-training assessment is the process of obtaining evidence in order to make judgements about the progress of learners towards attainment of the learning objectives of an educational programme. Methods used to collect such data include formal tests, assignments, projects, class presentations and reports. Evidence may be provided by self, peer or supervisors. Feedback should be given to learners for all in-training assessment.

    Performance assessment is the assessment of practice in the real world. It reflects what professionals actually do, rather than what they can do under examination conditions, which is **assessment of competence**.

    Summative assessment is assessment designed to make a decision about the suitability of a candidate to proceed to the next stage (e.g. from year 1 to year 2 or from learner to 'qualified'). The nature of summative assessment may vary according to how high the stakes are. For the RACGP training programme, the College examination is the summative assessment.

Behavioural anchors are the descriptors provided to guide the scoring of a rating scale. Ideally they are detailed enough to allow the scorer to clearly differentiate performance being observed. For example, instead of 'excellent' to describe a score of 10 (out of 10) for gathering information in a clinical history, the description might be 'Gathers all possible information, including relevant past history'.

Checklist is an aid to structured scoring of answers. They vary from long detailed subcomponents of desirable responses to more global categories.

Compensation of scores across subtests is the ability for strong performance in one subtest to make up for weak performance in another. This acknowledges that performance should be measured as a whole, rather than as scores of individual test methods.

Competencies are individual aspects of competence that can be learned and assessed.

Curriculum is a statement about the content of knowledge included in a training course and the process by which it will be learned. It is usually expressed in terms of learning objectives, domains and competencies. Ideally, a curriculum includes details of how learners will be assessed and how the training course will be evaluated.

Domains or areas of competence are conceptual groupings of competencies that organise and represent the main concepts incorporating the knowledge, skills and attitudes required for practice.

Error: Assessment error is the term that acknowledges the inherent errors associated with any measurement.

Evaluation is measurement against a standard for a defined purpose. In education, this usually means measurement of the extent to which educational objectives have been achieved, and in the real world we must evaluate in situations where there are no definite standards. In the context of assessment, it means the collection of information needed to make a judgement about the reliability, validity, educational impact and efficiency of the assessment.

Hurdles are assessments that must be completed prior to taking summative assessment. These are ideal for assessing components of competence that are not easily measured by formal test methods.

Learning objectives are clear, measurable statements about the expected educational outcomes of a training course.

Marking key is a structured 'ideal' answer to test items. It usually includes allocation of marks for parts of answers and should be prepared when the question or item is designed.

Objective Structured Clinical Examination (or Assessment) – OSCE (or OSCA) is an assessment format that combines several test methods, as appropriate for more integrated measurement of a range of competencies, particularly clinical and communication skills. It is not in itself a test method.

Psychometrics is the measurement of human behaviour and attributes. Complex methods are often used to achieve this. Psychometricians are those who practise the art.

Rating scale is an aid to structured scoring of answers, usually applied to clinical and communication skills assessments. There are two kinds: a semantic differential scale (very poor – poor – borderline – good – very good) and Likert scales (1–2–3–4–5). Different rating scales have unique measurement properties that need to be considered when combining scores of individual subtests.

> **Global rating scale** is a simple, often one-line scale that asks raters to assess overall performance. With experienced examiners, this is as reliable as more detailed methods.

Recognition of prior learning is where prior learning and clinical experiences are assessed as being relevant and valuable to the current course, and some credit (usually time or specific modules) is granted.

Reliability of an assessment is the extent to which assessment results can be repeated on more than one occasion – the consistency of assessment.

> **Inter-rater reliability** concerns the consistency of measures by more than one observer.

> **Reliability coefficients** are a statistical method of producing a score between 0 and 1 that indicates the reliability of the assessment. In general, a score of 0.8

or more is regarded as acceptable. The most common reliability coefficients are *generalisability coefficients*, which allow sources of error to be identified as a guide to improving reliability.

   Test–retest reliability concerns the consistency of assessment scores when the same candidates face the same assessment on two or more occasions.

Sampling of individual test items should be done randomly from an assessment blueprint. Random sampling works better with a larger bank of potential items. Stratified sampling is where items are sampled from within groupings with particular characteristics, such as domains, age groups, diagnoses, etc.

Standard Error of Measurement (S_E) is a statistical way of recognising both systematic and random error in measurement. It is derived by calculating the formula $S_E = S_x\sqrt{1-r}$, where S_x is the standard deviation and r is the test score reliability (e.g. Cronbach's *alpha*).

Standard setting is a process by which pass scores for each item and each test are determined on the basis of required level of performance, without reference to scores of candidates. Ideally, individual items have model, scored answers developed at the time of writing and agreed to by some sort of consensus process.

   Criterion-referenced (absolute standard) assessment. An external process that determines estimates of candidate performance and sets the passing score. As a result, the proportion of candidates passing may vary.

   Norm-referenced (relative standard) assessment. The performance of an individual is measured against the performance of the group as a whole. As an example, a pass score may be set at 50% or by reference to mean scores for the group, rather than an external standard. Hence there tends to be a relatively fixed proportion of passes and failures.

Test battery is a combination of more than one test method and/or format, or subtests.

Test blueprint is a structured method to guide sampling of individual test items. Wherever possible, this should reflect the universe of potential competencies and be based on data that define those competencies, e.g. morbidity, age and gender data on presentations to general practice, domains of competence.

Test format is an assessment mode, e.g. written test, clinical test. There are several possible *test methods* within formats, such as MCQ and Modified Essay Questions (written) and simulated patient encounter and observed physical examination (clinical). Each test method has strengths and weaknesses and may assess particular components better than others.

Triangulation is the measurement of an attribute, or group of attributes, from more than one perspective. Similar findings from different perspectives strengthen each other and the overall result.

Universe of competence includes all possible competencies in all domains. This may include attributes that are not easily assessed.

Validity of a test is the extent to which it measures what it is intended to measure.

   Construct validity is the extent to which assessment instruments measure the behaviours intended to be measured.

   Content validity is the extent to which a test measures the relevant clinical content.

Criterion validity is the extent to which measurements agree with those of an accepted 'standard' test.

Face validity is the extent to which a test appears to be acceptable to stakeholders.

Predictive validity is the extent to which test performance predicts changes in behaviour (or other attributes) in the future.

Weighting of particular aspects of competence may be applied if there is evidence and agreement that these are more important than other aspects or components. Methods of weighting include over-sampling, awarding higher scores or creating hurdles.

Puzzles of clinical reasoning revealed

(a) Hypothetico-deductive 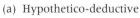   (b) Pattern matching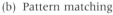

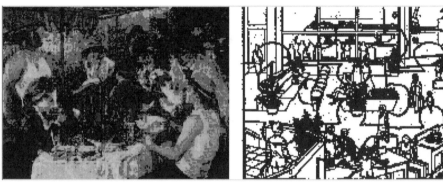

Figure 2.3 Models of clinical reasoning – full images.

References

Balint M (1986) *The Doctor, The Patient and The Illness*. Edinburgh: Churchill Livingstone.

Bligh J (1993) The S-SLDRS: a short questionnaire about self-directed learning. *Postgraduate Education for General Practice*. **4**: 255–6.

Brennan TA *et al.* (1991) Hospital characteristics associated with adverse events and substandard care. *JAMA*. **265**: 3265–9.

Consumer Health Forum, Commonwealth of Australia (1996) *Integrating Consumer Views About Quality in General Practice*. Canberra: Australian Government Publishing Service.

Cusimano MD (1996) Standard setting in medical education. *Academic Medicine*. **71** (Suppl.): S112–20.

Deveugele M *et al.* (2004) Is the communication behaviour of GPs during the consultation related to the diagnosis. A cross sectional study in six European countries. *Patient Educ Counselling*. **54**: 227–33.

Diamond MR, Kamien M, Sim MB and Davis J (1995) A critical incident study of general practice trainees in their basic general practice term. *Medical Journal of Australia*. **162**: 321–4.

Donabedian A (1988) The quality of care: how can it be assessed? *Journal of the American Medical Association*. **260**: 1743–8.

Foulkes J *et al.* (1994) Combining components of competence. In: Newble D, Jolly B and Wakeford R (eds) *The Certification and Recertification of Doctors*. Cambridge: Cambridge University Press.

Greco M, Francis W, Buckley J, Brownlea A and McGovern J (1998) Real patient evaluation of communication skills teaching for GP registrars. *Family Practice*. **15** (1): 51–7.

Greenhalgh T (1997a) How to read a paper: getting your bearings (deciding what the paper is about). *British Medical Journal*. **315**: 243–6.

Greenhalgh T (1997b) How to read a paper: assessing the methodological quality of published papers. *British Medical Journal*. **315**: 305–8.

Greenhalgh T (1997c) Papers that report drug trials. *British Medical Journal*. **315**: 480–3.

Greenhalgh T (1997d) Papers that report diagnostic or screening tests. *British Medical Journal*. **315**: 540–1.

Grol R and Lawrence M (1995) *Quality Improvement by Peer Review*. Oxford General Practice Series 32. Oxford: Oxford University Press.

Harden RM and Davis M (1995) The core curriculum with options or special study modules. *Medical Teacher*. **17**: 125–48.

Hays RB (1989) The diagnostic content of consultations collected for teaching purposes. *Australian Family Physician*. **1** (7): 846–51.

Hays RB (1990a) Content validity of a rating scale for general practice consultations. *Medical Education*. **2** (2): 110–16.

Hays RB (1990b) Self-evaluation of videotaped consultations. *Teaching and Learning in Medicine*. **2** (4): 232–6.

Hays RB and Wellard R (1998) In-training assessment in postgraduate training for general practice. *Medical Education*. **32**: 307–12.

Hays RB *et al.* (2002a) Is insight important? Measuring the capacity to change. *Medical Education*. **36**: 965–71.

Hays RB *et al.* (2002b) A performance assessment module for experienced general practitioners. *Medical Education*. **36**: 258–60.

Hobma SO *et al.* (2004) Setting the standard for performance assessment of doctor–patient communication in general practice. *Medical Education.* **38**: 1244–52.

Honey P and Mumford A (1986) *Manual of Learning Styles.* Maidenhead: Honey.

Howard K and Sharp JA (1994) *The Management of a Student Research Project.* Aldershot: Gower Publishing.

Larkins SL *et al.* (2004) Isolation, flexibility and change in vocational training for general practice: personal and educational problems experienced by general practice registrars in Australia. *Family Practice.* **21**: 559–66.

Lewis AP and Bolden KJ (1989) General practitioners and their learning styles. *Journal of the Royal College of General Practitioners.* **13**: 187–9.

Miller GE (1990) The assessment of clinical skills/competence/performance. *Academic Medicine.* **65** (Suppl.): 563–7.

Murray E, Todd C and Modell M (1997) Can general internal medicine be taught in general practice? An evaluation of the University College of London model. *Medical Education.* **31**: 369–74.

Pendleton D, Schofield T, Tate P and Havelock P (1984) *The Consultation: an approach to teaching and learning.* Oxford: Oxford University Press.

Pitts J, Percy D and Coles C (1995) Evaluating teaching. *Education for General Practice.* **6**: 13–18.

Rethans JJ (1996) Methods of quality assessment in general practice. *Family Practice.* **13**: 468–76.

Rethans JJ, Martin E and Metsemakers J (1994) To what extent do clinical notes by general practitioners reflect actual performance? A study using simulated patients. *British Journal of General Practice.* **44**: 153–6.

Sackett D, Richardson WS, Rosenberg W and Haynes RB (1997) *Evidence-based Medicine.* London: Pearson Professional Publishing.

Sen Gupta TK, Wallace DA, Clark SL and Bannon G (1998) Videoconferencing: practical advice on implementation. *Australian Journal of Rural Health.* **6**: 2–4.

Silagy C and Haines A (1998) *Evidence-based Practice in Primary Care.* London: BMJ Books.

Streiner DL and Norman GR (1993) *Health Measurement Scales. A practical guide to their development and use.* Oxford: Oxford University Press.

Wilson RM *et al.* (1999) An analysis of the causes of adverse events from the Quality in Australian Healthcare Study. *Medical Journal of Australia.* **170**: 411–15.

Some suggestions for a teaching practice library

The following items have been selected particularly for their relevance to teaching, rather than to clinical practice.

Books

General Medical Council (2002) *Good Medical Practice*. London: GMC. (Most Medical Councils have similar editions.)
The practice should have a copy on hand of the local Medical Council's views on the desired end product of the training.

Hall M, Dwyer D and Lewis T (1999) *The GP Training Handbook* (3e). Oxford: Blackwell Science.

Jones R, Britten N, Culpepper L *et al.* (eds) (2004) *Oxford Textbook of Primary Medical Care.* Oxford: Oxford University Press.
Now more or less the international standard for a comprehensive textbook of primary care. While more oriented to the UK system, it also includes sections written for several other nations to explain the local differences in primary care.

McWhinney IR (1997) *A Textbook of Family Medicine* (2e). Oxford: Oxford University Press.
Still arguably the best presentation of the underlying philosophy of general practice.

Mohanna K, Wall D and Chambers R (2004) *Teaching Made Easy*. Oxford: Radcliffe Publishing.
Perhaps it is not so easy to do well, but this book provides further educational theoretical context to day-to-day teaching.

Murtagh J (1994) *General Practice*. Sydney: McGraw Hill Book Company.
A comprehensive presentation of general practice, mostly from an Australian perspective, but it travels well to other nations.

Neighbour R (1987) *The Inner Consultation*. London: Kluwer Academic Publishers.
Arguably a classic, an interesting although rather unusual approach.

Nyman KC (1996) *Successful Consulting*. Melbourne: Royal Australian College of General Practitioners.
Presents what has been distilled from 'sitting in' on several hundred consultations.

Pendleton D, Schofield T, Tate P and Havelock P (1984) *The Consultation: an approach to teaching and learning*. Oxford: Oxford University Press.

Silagy C and Haines A (eds) (1998) *Evidence-based Practice in Primary Care*. London: BMJ Books.

Stewart M, Brown JB, Weston WW, McWhinney IR, McWilliam CL and Freeman TR (1995) *Patient-centred Medicine: transforming the clinical method*. Thousand Oaks, CA: Sage Publications, Inc.

For rural practices

Hays RB (2002) *Practising Rural Medicine in Australia*. Melbourne: Eruditions Publishing.
Deals with the personal and professional challenges encountered in rural practice; mainly for registrars. Australian context, but generic messages.

Wilkinson D, Hays R, Strasser R and Worley P (2004) *The Handbook of Rural Medicine in Australia*. Melbourne: Oxford University Press.
Simple, practical textbook mainly aimed at medical student level. Australian context, but would be relevant in nations with similar rural environments.

Journals to buy or browse regularly

Education for Primary Care. Radcliffe Publishing, Oxford.
Very practical, aimed at those who teach in general practice, mostly at the vocational training level. Most relevant to the broader primary care context found in the UK.
Medical Teacher. Radcliffe Publishing, Oxford.
Practical, wide range of topics, more relevant to UK and undergraduate contexts.
Teaching and Learning in Medicine. Lawrence Erlbaum Associates, New York.
Stronger research base, covering both undergraduate and postgraduate issues.
Medical Education. Blackwell Science, Oxford.
Strong research base. Includes reports on innovations, book reviews and short reports covering all aspects of medical education.
Academic Medicine. American Association of Medical Colleges, Philadelphia.
Strong research/methodology base, oriented towards North American and mostly medical school contexts, but some useful articles, such as reviews of new books and educational software.

Websites

http://www.

Net address	Theme
bmj.com	*British Medical Journal*
mja.com.au	*Medical Journal of Australia*
blacksci.co.uk	The journal *Medical Education*
cme.net.au	Rural continuing medical education network
racgp.org.au	Royal Australian College of General Practitioners resource centre
rcgp.org.uk	Royal College of General Practitioners resource centre
rnzcgp.org.au	Royal New Zealand College of General Practitioners resource centre
aaagp.org.au	Australian Association for Academic General Practice
dundee.ac.uk/meded/amee	Association for Medical Education in Europe
aamc.org	American Association of Medical Colleges
asme.org.uk	Association for the Study of Medical Education
stfm.org	Society of Teachers of Family Medicine (US)

All medical schools have their own websites. Check on the address for the medical school with which you are affiliated.

Index

Page numbers in *italics* refer to tables or figures.